case studies *in* ALLIED HEALTH ETHICS

case studies *in* ALLIED HEALTH ETHICS

Robert M. Veatch
Director, Joseph and Rose Kennedy Institute of Ethics
Georgetown University

Harley E. Flack
President, Wright State University

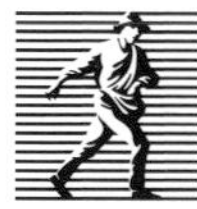

PRENTICE HALL, Upper Saddle River, NJ 07458

ublication Data

Case Studies in Allied Health Ethics / Robert M. Veatch, Harley E. Flack
p. cm.
Includes bibliographical references and index
ISBN 0-8359-4995-8
1. Medical ethics—Case studies. 2. Allied health personnel—Professional ethics—Case studies. I. Harley E. Flack.
R724, V398 1997
174' .2—DC20 96–3696
CIP

Editorial/production supervision and interior design: *Carol Lavis*
Director of Production and Manufacturing: *Bruce Johnson*
Managing Editor: *Patrick Walsh*
Acquisitions Editor: *Barbara Krawiec*
Manufacturing Buyer: *Ilene Sanford*
Marketing Manager: *Judith Streger*
Formatter: *Stephen J. Hartner*
Cover design: *Bruce Kenselaar*

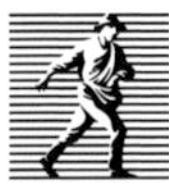

Printed in the United States of America

10 9 8 7 6 5 4 3 2 1

ISBN 0-8359-4995-8

Prentice-Hall International (UK) Limited, *London*
Prentice-Hall of Australia Pty. Limited, *Sydney*
Prentice-Hall Canada Inc., *Toronto*
Prentice-Hall Hispanoamericana, S.A., *Mexico*
Prentice-Hall of India Private Limited, *New Delhi*
Prentice-Hall of Japan, Inc., *Tokyo*
Simon & Schuster Asia Pte. Ltd., *Singapore*
Editora Prentice-Hall do Brasil, Ltda., *Rio de Janeiro*

CONTENTS

CASES

PREFACE

Providing health care increasingly requires ethical choices. Allied health personnel, who constitute the largest segment of the health care system in the United States, are by no means exempt from these choices. The day is gone—if, indeed, it ever existed—when the members of the health care team who are not physicians could consider themselves to be doing their jobs adequately if they simply followed orders.

As do all professions, the allied health professions impose ethical standards and obligations on their practitioners. While the specific ethical responsibilities will vary from one allied health profession to another, there are many problems that are shared.

To begin, virtually any allied health professional may be asked by a physician, other health care provider, or patient to engage in actions that are not consistent with the allied health professional's own conscience. The respiratory care therapist may be asked to discontinue providing maintenance of a ventilator; the medical records professional may be asked to conceal controversial portions of a record from a patient, professional colleagues, or public officials; a dietitian may receive a request for hyperalimentation for a patient who the dietitian knows opposes the procedure; a radiographer may recognize that the decision to execute an intricate surgery is based, in large part, on an x-ray that is of questionable quality.

Other allied health professionals may be held accountable for their actions when their professional associations have codes calling for certain kinds of conduct. These, at least, put the profession on record as viewing the work of its members as people responsible for their actions. The codes may conflict, however, with the instructions of the physician, the wishes of the patient, or the conscience of the individual care giver. The codes of the various allied health professions, as we shall see, may actually come in conflict with one another. The code of the physician assistant, for example, specifically authorizes breaking confidences under certain circumstances. So did the code of the occupational therapist until its most recent revision, but the conditions under which confidences could have been broken were different in the two groups. Meanwhile, the code of the American Society for Medical Technology offers no exceptions to the confidentiality principle. Clearly, ethical problems are going to arise when one allied health professional interacts with another from a different group, even if the individual happens to agree completely with the ethical norms of his or her own profession.

The physical therapist's opinion about divulging to a patient the truth of the patient's terminal prognosis may be contrary to the occupational therapist's desire to avoid the issue. Likewise, the speech pathologist may feel obliged to reveal that the burns on a neurologically damaged patient are the result of negligence on the part of a physical therapist who administered heat treatment for too long a period of time.

Every member of an allied health profession is constantly making ethical choices. Sometimes those choices are dramatic, life-and-death decisions, but often they will be more subtle, less conspicuous choices that are nonetheless important. One way to see the implication of these choices is to look at the experiences of one's colleagues, to listen to their stories and the kinds of choices they have had to make in situations like the ones typically faced by members of the allied health professions. This volume is a collection of those situations. It is, we believe, the best way to study the biomedical ethics of the allied health professions.

Articulating a definition of allied health is a difficult, if not impossible, task. According to Farber, McTernan, and Hawkins, as many as 85 distinct and different fields employing as many as 2.5 million individuals can be included within the scope of allied health personnel.[1] Arriving at a common definition is made more difficult because of differences that exist with several important policy-related characteristics of allied health professions or personnel, for example, the level of autonomy, dependence on technology, degree of regulation, and nature and extent of education/training.

According to the Institute of Medicine (IOM) study report,[2] several definitions of allied health have been advanced including that of the Committee on Allied Health Education and Accreditation and the National Commission on Allied Health Education (1980). Their definitions are, respectively,

> a large cluster of health care related professions and personnel whose functions include assisting, facilitating, or complementing the work of physicians and other specialists in the health care system, and who choose to be identified as "allied health personnel."

> all health personnel working toward the common goal of providing the best possible service in patient care and health promotion.

Although there may be significant disagreement regarding the definition of allied health, many do concur that the allied health professions are an indispensable albeit often unrecognized resource in the health care system.

In preparing this manuscript, collecting case studies from 85 allied health fields was both impractical and undesirable. Hence, one of the first problems encountered was to decide which allied health fields to include in developing case studies. The criteria we employed parallel to a large extent those used in selecting allied fields that are the focus of the 1988 IOM study report.

Autonomy

Allied health fields that have a relatively high level of independence in the clinical setting were selected. In some instances, for example, physical therapy and dietetics, allied health professionals now attract their own patients and therefore practice almost exclusively autonomously.

Degree of Regulation

For this text, allied health personnel who are regulated by licensure, certification, or register with a governmental agency were selected. Such allied health fields, of course, also have their own statements of professional standards of practice and behavior.

Dependence on Technology

The allied health fields that are highlighted in this volume have a significant dependence on technology. While concurring with the IOM hypothesis that "those who become broadly involved in one or more technologies are less vulnerable to obsolescence," they are at the same time more vulnerable perhaps to encountering ethical dilemmas in their practice. As will be seen later in this volume, numerous ethical dilemmas arise as allied health personnel employ technology in patient care and research.

Given these criteria, the nine allied health fields selected for focus in this book are as follows:

1. Radiography/Radiologic Technology

In 1920, a handful of x-ray technicians formed the American Association of Radiological Technicians in Chicago. This was 25 years after Wilhelm Roentgen discovered x-rays. As of 1986, according to the Bureau of Health Professions, there were 143,000 radiologic health services workers in the United States.

2. Clinical Laboratory Technology

In 1987, there were 37,271 technicians and 172,214 technologists, according to the American Society of Clinical Pathologists. The first clinical laboratory was established at the University of Michigan in 1875. Clinical laboratory work began with physicians and spread to nonphysicians as the field grew and became more complex and time consuming.

3. Dietetics

The American Dietetics Association (ADA) was established in 1918. Fifty-one years later (1969), the ADA developed a registry of dietitians. Dietetics or nutritionists number approximately 44,000 (ADA members).

4. Physical Therapy

In the face of World War I, 800 reconstruction aides were trained to work in army hospitals. From these aides, the American Women's Physical Therapeutic Association was formed in 1920. This association evolved to the American Physical Therapy Association, which, in 1986, estimated there to be 66,000 licensed physical therapists in the United States.

5. Respiratory Care

In 1986, the Bureau of Labor Statistics estimated that over 56,000 respiratory therapists were employed in this country. This field of allied health developed and grew after World War II. The American Association for Respiratory Care is the professional organization for respiratory care practitioners.

6. Occupational Therapy

Working in such settings as rehabilitation and psychiatric hospitals, schools, and nursing and home health agencies, occupational therapists have evolved since their beginnings in 1906 when the first training course was established in Boston. In 1987, there were 27,000 occupational therapists who were members of the American Occupational Therapy Association.

7. Physician Assistants

Physician assistants are among the newest allied health personnel. Developing during and immediately after the war in Vietnam, paramedics evolved through the acquisition of more formal training/education. Today, there are 24,000 practicing physician assistants who provide important services in our health care system.

8. Health Information Management

This field of allied health employed 8,240 registered health information management administrators and 14,000 accredited record technicians in 1987. The American Health Information Management Association is regarded as the national organization. Commencing their work in 1897, medical records personnel provide indispensable services.

9. Speech-Language Pathology and Audiology Services

The final allied health field to be included in this book is speech-language pathology and audiology. In 1986 there were 45,000 jobs for audiologists and speech-language pathologists. The professional organization for these personnel is American Academy of Speech Correction.

In all, the nine allied health fields outlined here employ more than 598,725 workers. The individuals who work in these nine fields constitute a significant force in the health care system. Taken together with the many other members of the health care team who daily face difficult moral situations, the instances wherein allied health personnel collectively have involvement in the value-based and ethical dimensions of health care are of such magnitude quantitatively and qualitatively that the exploration of issues contained in this volume is long overdue.

This collection of cases is based on real-life experiences of practicing allied health personnel. We have modified details to protect anonymity and provide greater clarity in presenting the ethical issues, but in each case some allied health professional has had to face the problems presented here. We are grateful to many informants who helped us by providing cases. Some are acknowledged in conjunction with the presentation of various cases. Others are acknowledged at the end of the volume. Still others have asked that we not reveal their identity in order to provide further protection of anonymity.

In addition to these informants who helped by providing case material, we also want to acknowledge the assistance of a number of others who provided research or clerical assistance including Irene McDonald, Carol Mason Spicer, Kier Olsen and William Stempsey, M.D., S.J., all of Georgetown University's Kennedy Institute of Ethics, Evelyn Vanaman of Rowan College of New Jersey and Linda Dull and Diane Barfield of Wright State University. While we appreciate their help, we are, of course, solely responsible for judgments contained in the volume.

ENDNOTES

1. Norman E. Farber, Edmund J. McTernan, and Robert O. Hawkins. *Allied Health Education.* (Springfield, IL: Thomas, 1989).
2. Institute of Medicine. Committee to Study the Role of Allied Health Personnel. *Allied Health Services.* (Washington, DC: National Academy Press, 1989).

INTRODUCTION

Four Questions of Ethics

As a field, biomedical ethics presents a fundamental problem. As a branch of applied ethics, biomedical ethics becomes interesting and relevant only when it abandons the ephemeral realm of theory and abstract speculation and gets down to practical questions raised by real, everyday problems of health and illness. Much of biomedical ethics, especially as practiced within the health professions, is indeed oriented to the practical questions of what should be done in a particular case. The allied health professions are, thus, case oriented. Yet if those who must resolve the ever-increasing ethical dilemmas in health care—including allied health professionals as well as patients, physicians, hospital administrators, and public policymakers—treat every case as something entirely fresh, entirely novel, they will have lost perhaps the best way of reaching solutions: to understand the general principles of ethics and face each new situation from a systematic ethical stance.

This is a volume of case studies in allied health ethics. It begins by recognizing the fact that one cannot consider any ethics, especially health care ethics, in the abstract. It is real-life, flesh-and-blood cases that raise fundamental ethical questions. It also recognizes that a general framework is needed from which to resolve the dilemmas of practicing one's profession. The cases in this volume are therefore organized in a systematic way. The chapters and issues within the chapters are arranged in order to work systematically through the questions of ethics. Since the main purpose of the book is to provide a collection of case studies from which may be built a more comprehensive scheme for health care ethics, the first few pages are addressed to the more theoretical issues. The object is to construct a framework of the basic questions in ethics that must be answered in any complete and systematic bioethical system.

Four fundamental questions must be answered in order to take a complete and systematic ethical position. Each question has several plausible answers, which have been developed over two thousand years of Western thought. For normal day-to-day decisions made by the allied health professional, it is not necessary to deal with each question. In fact, to do so would paralyze the decision maker. Most decisions are quite ordinary—deciding the diet for a patient, the proper exercises in physical therapy, or the exposure levels for an x-ray—and do not always demand full ethical analysis. Other decisions, as in the case of emergency intervention, are not ordinary at all. Still, in both the ordinary and emergency situations, it is possible only to act without being immobilized by the ethical and other value problems because some general rules or guidelines have emerged from previous experience and reflection. If ethical conflict is serious enough, it will be necessary to deal, at least implicitly, with all four fundamental questions of ethics.

WHAT MAKES RIGHT ACTS RIGHT?

At the most general level, which ethicists call the level of *metaethics*, the first question is: What makes right acts right? What are the meaning and justification of ethical statements?

It may not at first be obvious what counts as an ethical problem for allied health professionals. They easily recognize the moral crisis in deciding to let an abnormal newborn die, in choosing which of two needy patients will get a heart transplant, in participating in a late-term abortion for what to the allied health professional seems like trivial reasons, or helping a terminally ill patient in pain end his life. These situations clearly seem to involve ethical problems. Yet it is not immediately evident why we call these problems ethical while others faced more commonly in the routine practice of health care are not.

To make ethical problems obvious, several steps should be followed:

1. *Distinguish between evaluative statements and statements presenting nonevaluative facts.* Ethics involves making evaluations; therefore, it is a normative enterprise. Moving from the judgment that we can do something to the one that we ought to do something involves incorporating a set of norms—of judgments of value, rights, duties, responsibilities, and the like. Thus, to be ethically responsible in health care, it is important to develop the ability to recognize evaluations as they are made.

> STEPS IN ANALYZING AN ETHICAL PROBLEM
>
> 1. Distinguish between evaluative statements and statements presenting nonevaluative facts.
> 2. Distinguish between moral and nonmoral evaluations.
> 3. Determine who ought to decide.

Terms Signaling Normative Evaluations		
Verbs	**Nouns**	**Adjectives**
Want	Benefit	Good
Desire	Harm	Bad
Prefer	Duty	Right
Should	Responsibility	Wrong
Ought	Right	Responsible
	Obligation	Fitting

To develop this ability, select an experience that, at first, seems to involve no particular value judgments. Begin describing what occurred and watch for evaluative words. Every time a word expressing value is encountered, note it. Among the words to watch for are verbs such as want, desire, prefer, should, or ought. The evaluations may also be expressed in nouns such as benefit, harm, duty, responsibility, right, or obligation or in related adjectives such as good and bad, right and wrong, responsible, fitting, and the like.

Sometimes the evaluations are expressed in terms that are not necessarily literal, direct expressions of evaluations but are clearly functioning as value judgments. The *Code of Ethics for the Profession of Dietetics* of the American Dietetic Association (ADA), for example, states that "The dietetic practitioner provides sufficient information to enable clients to make their own informed decisions."[1] By this statement, the ADA could be describing the facts about the way all dietitians behave. Obviously it is not, however. Rather, it is saying that the dietitian ought to provide this information and that the good dietitian does so provide them.

2. *Distinguish between moral and nonmoral evaluations.* This process can be much harder, since often the difference cannot be discerned from the language itself. If one says that the dietitian did a good job of informing the patient about the reasons for instituting parenteral nutrition and the alternatives, the statement could express many kinds of evaluations. It could mean that the dietitian did a good job legally, that the dietitian fulfilled the law. It could mean that the dietitian did a good job psychologically, that the job was done in a way that produced a good psychological impact on the patient. It could mean that the dietitian did a good job technically, that every relevant piece of information was conveyed accurately. Or it could mean that the dietitian did a good job ethically, that the dietitian did what was morally required. Conceivably, a good explanation in one of these senses could simultaneously be a bad explanation in some other sense.

Sometimes value judgments in health care simply express nonmoral evaluations. Saying that the patient ate well does not express a moral evaluation of the way the patient consumed the food. Saying that another day's hospitalization for the patient will be good means only that the patient will be helped physically or psychologically, not morally. Even these apparently nonmoral judgments about benefits and harms, however, may quickly lead one into the sphere of ethics. When the client's judgment of what will be beneficial, for example, differs from the health professional's judgment, specific ethical dilemmas may emerge. A health professional who is committed morally to doing what will benefit the client will choose one course, while the one who is committed to preserving client autonomy may reluctantly choose the other.

Ethical or moral evaluations are judgments of what is good or bad, right or wrong, having certain characteristics that separate them from other evaluations such as aesthetic judgments, personal preferences, beliefs, or matters of taste. The difference between the evaluations lies in the grounds on or the reasons for which the evaluations are being made.[2]

Moral evaluations possess certain characteristics. They are evaluations of human actions, practices, or character traits rather than inanimate objects such as paintings or architectural structures. Not all evaluations of human actions are moral evaluations, however. We may say that the medical records librarian is a good administrator or a good teacher without making a moral evaluation. To be considered moral, an evaluation must have additional characteristics. Three characteristics are often mentioned as the distinctive characteristics of moral evaluations. First, the evaluations must be ultimate. They must have a certain preemptive quality, meaning that other values or human ends cannot, as a rule, override them.[3] Second, they must possess universality. Moral evaluations are thought of as reflecting a standpoint that applies to everyone. They are evaluations that everyone in principle ought to be able to make and understand (even if some in fact do not do so).[4] Finally, many add a third, more material, condition: that moral evaluations must treat the good of everyone alike. They must be general in the sense that they avoid giving a special place to one's own welfare. They must have an other-regarding focus or, at least, consider one's own welfare no more important than that of others.[5]

CHARACTERISTICS OF MORAL EVALUATIONS

1. The evaluations must be ultimate.
2. The evaluations must possess universality.
3. The evaluations must treat the good of everyone alike.

Moral judgments possessing these characteristics can sometimes conflict with one another. Conflicts over whether the health care provider ought to care for a client in the way thought to be most beneficial or most respecting of the client's autonomy (even though harm may result) can involve conflicts between moral characteristics. If that is the case, any decision in clinical practice that involves a conflict over values potentially involves a moral conflict. The care giver may be faced with the choice between preserving the client's welfare or someone else's. The provider may have to choose whether to keep a promise of confidentiality or provide needed assistance for a client even though a confidence would have to be broken. The care giver may have to decide whether to protect the interests of colleagues or of the institution and whether to serve future patients by striking for better conditions or serve present patients by refusing to strike. These are moral conflicts faced by health care professionals. Chapter 1 presents a series of cases where both moral and nonmoral evaluations are made in what appear to be quite ordinary health care situations faced by various allied health professionals. The main task is to discern the value dimensions and to separate them from the physiological, psychological, and other facts.

3. *Determine who ought to decide.* A closely related problem that depends on the question of what makes right acts right is the question: Who ought to decide? This is the focus of Chapter 2. Having learned to recognize the difference between the factual and evaluative dimensions of a case in health care ethics, one will constantly encounter the problem of who ought to decide or where the locus of decision making ought to rest. The answer will depend, of course, on deciding from where morals come. Chapter 2 presents cases considering a range of sources of moral authority, from the various allied health professional organizations, health care institutions, patients, families, physicians, and administrators to professional committees and the general public.

The choice among these decision makers depends, at least in part, on what it is that ethical terms mean, or more generally, what it is that makes right acts right. Several answers to this question have been offered. One answer recognizes that different societies seem to reach different conclusions about whether a given act is right or wrong. From this perspective, to say that an act is morally right means nothing more than that it is in accord with the values of the group to which the speaker belongs or simply that it is approved by the speaker's group. This position, called *social relativism,* explains rightness or wrongness on the basis of whether the act fits with social customs, mores, and folkways of the group. One problem with this view is that it seems to make sense to say that some act is morally wrong even though it is approved by the speaker's group. That would be impossible if moral judgments were based simply on the values of the speaker's group.

A second answer to the question of what makes right acts right attempts to correct this problem. According to this position, to say that an act is right means that it is approved by the speaker. This position, called *personal relativism,* reduces ethical meaning to personal preference. Of course, according to this position, behavior thought to be immoral by some is approved by others. Some say that the reason this can happen is that moral judgments are merely expressions of the speaker's preference.

Such differences in judgment, however, may have another explanation than that ethical terms refer to the speaker's own preferences. Those disagreeing might simply not be working with the same facts. To claim that two people are in moral disagreement simply because the same act is seen as right by one person or group and wrong by another requires proof that both see the facts in the same way. Differences of circumstances or belief about the facts could easily account for many moral differences.

In contrast with social and personal relativism, there is a third group of answers to the question of what makes right acts right. These positions, collectively called *universalism* or sometimes *absolutism,* hold that, in principle, acts that are called morally right or wrong are right or wrong independent of social or personal views. Certainly some choices merely involve personal taste: flavors of ice cream or hair lengths vary from time to time, place to place, and person to person. But these are matters of preference, not morality. No one considers the choice of vanilla morally right and chocolate morally wrong. But other evaluations appeal beyond the standards of social and personal taste to a more ultimate or universal frame of reference. When these are concerned with acts or character traits—as opposed to, say, paintings or music—they are thought of as moral evaluations.

However, the nature of the universal standard is often disputed. For the theologically oriented, it may be a single divine standard as we see in the monotheistic religions. According to this view, calling it right to disconnect a respirator keeping alive a terminally ill, comatose patient is to say that God would approve of the act or that it is in accord with His will. This position is sometimes called *theological absolutism* or *theological universalism.*

Still another view among universalists takes empirical observation as the model. The standard in this case is nature or external reality. The problem of knowing whether an act is right or wrong is then the problem of knowing what is in nature. *Empirical absolutism,* as the view is sometimes called, sees the problem of knowing right and wrong as analogous to knowing scientific facts.[6] While astronomers try to discern the real nature of the universe of stars and chemists the real nature of atoms as ordered in nature, ethics, according to this view, is an effort to discern rightness and wrongness as ordered in nature. The position sometimes takes the form of a natural law position. As with the physicist's law of gravity, moral laws are thought to be inexplicably rooted in nature. Natural law positions may be secular or may have a theological foundation such as in the ethics of Thomas Aquinas and traditional Catholic moral theology.

Still another form of universalism or absolutism rejects both the theological and the empirical models. It supposes that right and wrong are not empirically knowable, but are nonnatural properties known only by intuition. Thus, the position is sometimes called *intuitionism* or *nonnaturalism*.[7] Although for the intuitionist or nonnaturalist right and wrong are not empirically knowable, they are still universal. All persons should in principle have the same intuitions about a particular act, provided they are intuiting properly. Still others, sometimes called rationalists, hold that reason can determine what is ethically required.[8]

There are additional answers to the question of what makes right acts right. One view—in various forms called *noncognitivism, emotivism,* or *prescriptivism,* which ascended to popularity during the mid-twentieth century—saw ethical utterances as evincing feelings about a particular act.[9] A full exploration of the answers to this most abstract of ethical questions is not possible here.[10] Ultimately, however, if an ethical dispute growing out of a case is serious enough and cannot be resolved at any other level, this question must be faced. If one says that it is wrong to tell the truth to a dying patient because it will produce anxiety, and another says that it is right to do so because consent to treatment is a moral imperative, some way must be found of adjudicating the dispute between the two views. One must ask what it is that makes right acts right, how conflicts can be resolved, what the final authority is for morality, and whose judgment about what is right should prevail.

WHAT KINDS OF ACTS ARE RIGHT?

A second fundamental question of ethics moves beyond determining what makes right acts right to ask: What kinds of acts are right? This is the realm of *normative ethics*. It questions whether there are any general principles or norms describing the characteristics that make actions right or wrong.

Two major schools of thought dominate Western normative ethics. One position looks at the consequences of acts; the other at what is taken to be inherent rights and wrongs. The first position claims that acts are right to the extent that they produce good consequences and wrong to the extent that they produce bad consequences. The key evaluative terms for this position, known in various forms as *utilitarianism* or *consequentialism,* are good and bad. The key is the consequences of ends of action. This is the position of John Stuart Mill and Jeremy Bentham, as well as of Epicurus,

St. Thomas Aquinas, and capitalist economics. St. Thomas, for example, argued that the first principle of the natural law is that "good is to be done and promoted and evil is to be avoided."[11]

Since St. Thomas stands at the center of the Roman Catholic natural law tradition, he illustrates that natural law thinking (which is one answer to the first question of what makes right acts right) is not incompatible with consequentialism. The two positions are answers to two different questions. While natural law thinkers are not always consequentialists, they can be.

Classical utilitarianism determines what kinds of acts are right by figuring the net of good consequences minus bad ones for each person affected and then adding up to find the total net good.[12] The certainty and duration of the benefits and harms are taken into account. This form of consequentialism is indifferent to who obtains the benefits and harms. Thus, if the total net benefits of providing respiratory care to a relatively healthy but powerful figure are thought to be greater than those of providing it to a sicker Medicare recipient, the healthy and powerful ought to be given the care without further ethical debate.

Traditional allied health ethics, like physician ethics, is oriented to benefiting patients. This tradition combines the utilitarian answer to the question of what kinds of acts are right with a particular answer to the question of to whom moral duty is owed. Loyalty is to the patient, and the goal is to what will produce the most benefit and avoid the most harm to the patient.

The ethics of the allied health professions have traditionally held that the care giver's primary commitment is to the patient's care and safety. Some interpret this as viewing protecting the patient from harm as being prior to benefiting the patient. As with the principle of physician ethics, *primum non nocere* or "first of all do no harm," this view gives special weight to avoiding harm over and above the weight given to goods that can be produced.

Among physicians the principle of doing no harm is often interpreted conservatively. When a potentially risky intervention is contemplated, harm may be avoided by refusing to intervene. That way, no harm is done (although the physician thereby avoids doing any good that the intervention could have brought). This form of consequentialism that gives priority to avoiding harm needs to be distinguished from classical utilitarianism in which goods and harms are counted equally in calculating the net benefit of an action.

These problems of the relation between classical utilitarianism (which counts benefits to all in society equally) and traditional health care ethics (which focuses on the individual patient and sometimes gives special weight to avoiding harms through the prescriptive duty of advocacy) are raised in the cases of Chapter 3.

Against these positions that are oriented to consequences, the other major group of answers to the question of what kinds of acts are right asserts that rightness and wrongness are inherent in the act itself independent of the consequences. These positions, collectively known as *formalism* or *deontologism*, hold that right- and wrong-making characteristics may be independent of consequences. Kant stated the position most starkly.[13]

Chapter 4 takes up problems of health care delivery and in doing so poses probably the most significant challenge to the consequentialist ethic. Today some of the most challenging ethical problems in health care arise in cases in which allied health professionals have so many demands placed on them that they cannot do everything they would like for all their patients. One approach is to simply determine which course of action will do the most good overall. That, however, could mean leaving some patients virtually without care. It seems unfair or unjust (even if it turns out to be efficient in maximizing the total good done). One principle that is sometimes thought to restrain the production of overall good is the principle of *justice*. Taken in the sense of fairness in distributing goods and harms, justice is held by many to be an ethical right-making characteristic even if the consequences are not the best.

The problem is whether it is morally preferable to have a higher net total of benefits in society even if unevenly distributed or to have a somewhat lower total good but to have that good more equally distributed. This issue will be the focus of the cases in Chapter 4. Utilitarians would argue that net benefits tend to be greater when benefits are distributed more evenly (because of decreasing marginal utility—that is, because the more benefits one possesses the less valuable each marginal additional benefit will be). They claim that the only reason to distribute goods, such as health care, evenly is to maximize the total good. On the other hand, the formalist who holds that justice is a right-making characteristic independent of utility does not require an item-by-item calculation of benefits and harms before concluding that the unequal distribution of goods is *prima facie* wrong, that is, wrong with regard to fairness.

Another major challenge to consequentialism comes from the principle of *autonomy*. Where classical utilitarianism demands noninterference with the autonomy of others in society only when this produces greater net benefits, Kantian formalism leads to the moral demand that persons and their beliefs be respected even if doing so will not produce good for the patient. The problems of conflict between the health care provider's nonconsequentialist duties to respect autonomy or self-determination of individual clients and consequentialist duties to produce benefit are discussed in Chapter 5.

Another ethical principle that many formalists hold to be independent of consequences is that of *veracity*, or truth-telling. As with the other principles, utilitarians argue that truth-telling is an operational principle designed to guarantee maximum benefit. When truth-telling does more harm than good, according to the utilitarians, there is no obligation to tell the truth. To them, telling the dying patient of his condition can be cruel and is, therefore, wrong. In contrast, to one who holds that truth-telling is a right-making ethical principle in itself, the problem of what the dying patient would be told is much more complex. This problem of what the patient would be told is the subject of Chapter 6.

Another principle that formalists may believe to be right-making independent of consequences is *fidelity*, especially the keeping of promises. Kant and others have held that breaking a promise is wrong, independent of the consequences. The utilitarian points out that breaking a promise often has bad consequences. If it were to become a usual practice, the act of promising itself would become useless. The formalist, although granting this danger, argues that there is something more intrinsically wrong in breaking a promise and that to know this one need not even go on to look at the consequences. The formalist might, with the utilitarian, grant that to look at consequences may reveal even more reasons to oppose promise-breaking, but this is not necessary to know that promise-breaking is *prima facie* wrong.

The provider-patient relationship can be viewed essentially as one involving promises or contracts or, to use a term with fewer legalistic implications, covenants. The relationship is founded on implied and sometimes explicit promises. One of these promises is that information disclosed in the provider-patient relationship is confidential, that it will not be disclosed by the health care provider without the patient's permission. The duty of confidentiality in ethics is really a specification of the principle of promise-keeping in ethics in general. In Chapter 7, cases present the various problems growing out of the ethical principle of fidelity.

The cases of Chapter 8 introduce a final principle that can be included in a general ethical system: the principle of *avoidance of killing*. All societies have some kind of prohibition on killing. The Buddhists make it one of their five basic precepts. Those in the Judeo-Christian tradition recognize it as one of the Ten Commandments. The moral foundation of the prohibition on killing is not always clear, however. For some people, those who base their ethic on doing good and avoiding evil, prohibiting killing is simply a rule summarizing the obvious conclusion that it usually harms people to kill them. If that is the full foundation of the prohibition on killing, then killing is just an example of a way that one can do harm.

This presents a problem, however. Many people believe they are aware of special cases where killing someone may actually do good, on balance. It will stop a greater evil that the one killed would otherwise have committed, or it will, in health care, possibly relieve a terminally ill patient of otherwise intractable pain. Is killing a human being always morally a characteristic of actions that tends to make them wrong, or is it wrong only when more harm than good results from the killing? For those who hold that killing is always a wrong-making characteristic, avoiding killing takes on a life as an independent principle, much like veracity or autonomy or fidelity. The cases of Chapter 8 explore these questions.

HOW DO RULES APPLY TO SPECIFIC SITUATIONS?

There is a third question in a general ethical stance. It stems from the fact that each case raising an ethical problem is in at least some ways situationally unique. The ethical principles of beneficence (producing benefit), justice, autonomy, veracity, fidelity, and avoidance of killing are extremely general. They are a small set of the most general right-making characteristics. The question is: How do the general principles apply to specific situations? As a bridge to the particular case, an intermediate, more specific set of rules is often used. These intermediate rules probably cause more problems in ethics than any other component of ethical theory. At the same time they are probably more helpful as guides to day-to-day behavior than anything else.

The problems arise in part because of a misunderstanding of the nature and function of these rules. Rules may have two functions. They may simply serve as guidelines summarizing conclusions we tend to reach in moral problems of a certain kind. When rules have this function of simply summarizing experience in similar situations of the past, they are called *rules of thumb, guiding rules,* or *summary rules.*

In contrast, rules may function to specify behavior that is required independent of individual judgment about a specific situation. The rules against abortion of a viable fetus or against killing a dying patient are examples of rules that are often directly linked to right-making characteristics. Sometimes this kind of rule is called a *rule of practice.* The rule specifies a practice that, in turn, is justified by the general principles. According to this rules-of-practice view, it is unacceptable to overturn a general practice simply because in a particular case the outcome would be better.

The conflict between those who take the rules more seriously and those who consider the situation to be the more critical determinant of moral rightness became one of the major ethical controversies in the mid-twentieth century. It is sometimes called the rules-situation debate.[14] At one extreme is the *rigorist* who insists that rules should never be violated. At the other is the *situationalist* who claims that rules never apply because every situation is unique. Probably both positions taken in the extreme lead to absurdity. Rigorists are immobilized when two of their rules conflict.

Situationalists are immobilized when they treat a situation as literally new with no help from past experience in similar if not identical situations.

This difference over how seriously rules should be taken cuts across the answers to the question of what kinds of action are right. One can be a utilitarian who assesses the consequences case by case or a "rule-utilitarian" who believes in the rules-of-practice view, holding that rules should govern individual moral choices, but that the rules should be chosen based on their expected consequences. Likewise, someone who is a deontologist—who believes there are certain inherent right-making characteristics of actions independent of the consequences—can either apply the general principles (such as autonomy or veracity) directly to individual situations or use them to generate a set of rules, which are then applied to individual cases.

The rules-situation debate does not lend itself to special cases grouped together. The problem arises continually throughout the cases in the volume. The final question, however, requires special chapters with cases selected to examine the problems raised.

WHAT OUGHT TO BE DONE IN SPECIFIC CASES?

After the determination of what makes right acts right, what kinds of actions are right, and how rules apply to specific situations, there are still left a large number of specific situations that make up the bulk of problems in health care ethics. The question remains, what ought to be done in a specific case or kind of case? Health care professionals, being particularly oriented to case problems, are given to organizing ethical problems around specific kinds of cases. Ethics too is sometimes divided into the problems of birth, life, and death.

The first two parts of this volume emphasize the overarching problems of how to relate facts to values, of who ought to decide, respecting autonomy, veracity, fidelity, avoidance of killing, and justice in health care delivery. These are among the larger questions of biomedical ethics. Part three shifts to cases involving specific problem areas. Cases in Chapter 9 raise the problems of abortion, sterilization, and conception control. Chapter 10 moves to the related problems of genetic counseling and engineering and of intervention in the prenatal period. The next chapters take up, in turn, the problems of mental health and the control of human behavior; human experimentation, consent, and the right to refuse medical treatment; and, finally, death and dying.

The answer to the question of what ought to be done in a specific case requires the integration of the answers to all of the other questions if a thorough analysis and justification is to be given. The first line of moral defense will probably be a set of moral rules and rights thought to apply to the case. In abortion, the right to control one's body and the right of the health care professional to practice his or her profession are pitted against the right to life. In human experimentation, the rules of informed consent pertain. Among the dying, rules about euthanasia conflict with the right to pursue happiness, and the right to refuse medical treatment conflicts with the rule that the health care provider ought to do everything possible to preserve life.

In many cases in which the tension between conflicting rules cannot be resolved, the analysis escalates from an issue of moral rules and rights to the higher, more abstract level of ethical principle. It must be determined, for example, whether informed consent is designed to maximize benefits to the experimental subject or to facilitate the subject's freedom of self-determination. It must also be explored whether harm to the patient justifies withholding information from the patient or whether the formalist truth-telling principles justifies disclosure.

The problem of what ought to be done in a specific case also requires a great deal of information other than the moral. It requires considerable empirical data. Value-relevant biological and psychological facts have developed around many case problems in biomedical ethics. The predictive capacity of a flat electroencephalogram may be important for the definition of death. The legal facts are relevant for the refusal of treatment. Basic religious and philosophical beliefs of the patient may be critical for resolving some cases in health care ethics. It is impossible to present all the relevant medical, genetic, legal, and psychological facts that are necessary for a complete analysis of any case, but it is possible to present the major facts required for understanding. Readers will have to supplement these facts for a fuller understanding of the cases, just as they will have to supplement their reading in ethical theory for a fuller understanding of the basic questions of ethics.

ENDNOTES

1. The American Dietetic Association, *Code of Ethics for the Profession of Dietetics and Review Process for Alleged Violations* (Chicago: ADA, 1991), p. 2.
2. William Frankena, *Ethics*, 2nd ed. (Englewood Cliffs, NJ: Prentice Hall, 1973), p. 62.
3. Tom L. Beauchamp and James F. Childress, eds., *Principles of Biomedical Ethics*, 2nd ed. (New York: Oxford University Press, 1983), p. 15.
4. Charles Fried, *Right and Wrong* (Cambridge, MA: Harvard University Press, 1978), p. 12

5. Beauchamp and Childress, eds., *Principles of Biomedical Ethics*, 2nd ed., pp. 16-17; John Rawls, *A Theory of Justice* (Cambridge, MA: Harvard University Press, 1971), pp. 131-136; Kurt Baier, *The Moral View* (New York: Random House, 1965), pp. 106-109.
6. Roderick Firth, "Ethical Absolutism and the Ideal Observer Theory," *Philosophy and Phenomonological Research*, Vol. 12 (1952), pp. 317-345; C. D. Broad, "Some Reflections on Moral-Sense Theories in Ethics," pp. 131-166 in *Proceedings, The Aristotelian Society*, 1944-1945.
7. W. D. Ross, *The Right and the Good* (Oxford: Oxford University Press, 1939).
8. Immanuel Kant, *Groundwork of the Metaphysic of Morals*, trans. H. J. Paton (New York: Harper and Row, 1964).
9. A. J. Ayer, *Language, Truth, and Logic* (London: Victor Gollancz, 1948); C. L. Stevenson, *Ethics and Language* (New Haven, CT: Yale University Press, 1944); R. M. Hare, *The Language of Morals* (Oxford: Clarendon Press, 1952).
10. For basic surveys of ethical theory, see Frankena, *Ethics*, and G. J. Warnock, *Contemporary Moral Philosophy* (New York: St. Martin's Press, 1967). For more detailed introductions, see Richard B. Brandt, *Ethical Theory: The Problems of Normative and Critical Ethics* (Englewood Cliffs, NJ: Prentice Hall, 1959); Tom L. Beauchamp, *Philosophical Ethics: An Introduction to Moral Philosophy* (New York: McGraw-Hill Book Company, 1982); Fred Feldman, *Introductory Ethics* (Englewood Cliffs, NJ: Prentice Hall, 1978); Paul W. Taylor, *Principles of Ethics: An Introduction* (Encino, CA: Dickenson, 1975). For readers containing classical sources, see Richard B. Brandt, *Value and Obligation: Systematic Readings in Ethics* (New York: Harcourt, Brace & World, 1961); A. I. Melden, ed., *Ethical Theories: A Book of Readings*, 2nd ed. (Englewood Cliffs, NJ: Prentice Hall, 1967).
11. Thomas Aquinas, *Summa Theologica*, I-II, A. 94, Art. 2., eds. Fathers of the English Dominican Province (London: R & T Washbourne, 1915).
12. Jeremy Bentham, "An Introduction to the Principles of Morals and Legislation," in *Ethical Theories: A Book of Readings*, ed. A. I. Melden (Englewood Cliffs, NJ: Prentice Hall, 1967), pp. 367-390,
13. Immanuel Kant, *Groundwork of the Metaphysic of Morals*, trans. H. J. Paton (New York: Harper and Row, 1964).
14. John Rawls, "Two Concepts of Rules," *The Philosophical Review*, Vol. 44 (1955), pp. 3-32; Joseph Fletcher, *Situation Ethics: The New Morality* (Philadelphia: Westminster Press, 1966); Paul Ramsey, *Deeds and Rules in Christian Ethics* (New York: Scribners, 1967); Michael D. Bayles, ed., *Contemporary Utilitarianism* (Garden City, NY: Doubleday, 1968).

PART I

ETHICS AND VALUES IN ALLIED HEALTH

CHAPTER 1

Values in Health and Illness

Allied health professionals sometimes approach case decisions believing that the decisions they have to make are primarily technical. In a sense they are correct. Health care today is scientifically complex. Often a great deal of technical information must be processed correctly by the allied health professional to deliver high-quality care.

Being technically knowledgeable is never going to be enough, however. Clinical decisions always involve more than knowledge of the scientific facts about the processes and likely outcomes of alternative interventions. They *always* involve a judgment by someone that the envisioned outcome is a good one, in fact that, all things considered, the mix of risks and benefits is better than with any alternative choice, including the choice of doing nothing at all.

These decisions always involve evaluative comparisons—whether options are better or worse. Sometimes, but not always, the evaluations are moral evaluations. They rely on judgments that a course is morally better or worse than others being considered. Often the comparisons may not involve moral evaluations at all. Rather, they will involve aesthetic, legal, or psychological judgments. They may simply be matters of personal preference of the individual making the judgment.

RECOGNIZING EVALUATIVE JUDGMENTS

The first task in studying cases in allied health ethics is learning to recognize how frequently these evaluative judgments occur in the various allied health professions. The cases of this chapter present rather routine situations faced by allied health practitioners. In each case the task will be to identify the value judgments and determine what kind of judgments they are. One should ask when evaluative judgments are necessary and whether they are moral evaluations or evaluations of some other kind.

One rather typical kind of value judgment arising repeatedly in the allied health professions is the judgment about whether a test should be repeated when the initial performance of the test was flawed in some way. The flaw can occur as a result of an equipment error and/or an error on the part of the allied health practitioner. In any case, some judgment has to be made about whether a repeated test is "worth it." Some might argue that this is a question to be asked of the physician who ordered the test, but even that way out of the problem requires some value judgments. In some cases, the problem with the original test may be so marginal that the allied health practitioner may not even be able to decide whether to call the problem to the physician's attention. In other cases, the allied health professional may correctly believe that he or she is more competent to assess the situation than the physician. In reading the first case, try to note all the points at which evaluative judgments are made by the radiographer or others.

CASE 1: Should the Flawed Test Be Repeated?

Lucy Forman had a chest x-ray series done in May in Dr. Raymond Hill's office as a part of a routine physical examination. Unfortunately, on the day the x-ray was taken, the office was backed up with a lot of patients and the film developer was not working properly. Consequently, Ms. Forman did not obtain the results of the x-ray series until one week later. When Dr. Hill received Ms. Forman's x-ray from the radiographer, he saw something in Ms. Forman's left lung that looked suspicious.

Dr. Hill consulted with the radiographer, Jean Johnson, who took the x-ray. Dr. Hill asked Ms. Johnson if in light of the problems that she had had with the developer, the x-ray should be repeated. Since Dr. Hill is an internist, he probably would send Ms. Forman to a specialist who practices out of the local hospital center regardless of the outcome of the second x-ray. There she would undoubtedly be given another series of x-rays. Jean Johnson is also aware that Ms. Forman is very concerned about the amount of radiation to which she is exposed. Since she is likely to be referred to a specialist, should she be given another x-ray in Dr. Hill's office is the question that Jean Johnson faces.*

Jean Johnson, the radiographer in this case, faces the initial question of whether to repeat the test that may have been flawed by a faulty film developer. Where are the evaluations that take place in the case as presented?

**This case was provided by Professor Patricia Bynum.*

Note, first, some clear value terms: *Should* the x-ray be repeated? The developer was not working properly. Something on the x-ray looked *suspicious*. These may appear to be technical matters, not matters of value judgment. Yet the fact that there are technical issues at stake does not rule out the presence of value judgments. To say that a developer is not working properly is to go beyond the factual realm in an important sense. The radiographer has certain expectations about how the developer will work. Some deviations from those expectations may be too minor to worry about; others may be thought to be serious; some, of course, could even be deviations for the better. To say that the developer is not working properly is to draw a line and claim not only that the deviation is a bad one, but that the line between acceptable and unacceptable performance has been crossed.

Likewise, to say that there is something that "looks suspicious" is to make a value judgment. We would not call an abnormally healthy looking lung "suspicious." Even if there is a tissue seen in the x-ray that is evaluated as problematic, it could be so minor that the physician or the radiographer would simply ignore it. This picture reveals something that is so bad that it is called "suspicious" (but not bad enough that it would be called "awful" or "disastrous"). All these are evaluative terms.

To reach an answer to Jean Johnson's question, some additional evaluations are necessary. Dr. Hill, the internist, could decide to keep Ms. Forman as a patient himself and not refer. Someone must make a judgment about whether the benefits to be gained by referral to a specialist justify the economic costs, inconvenience, and other reasons not to refer.

Underlying all these evaluations is the question of how to evaluate the radiation risks. Ms. Forman has already had one x-ray series. She is a candidate for another from Dr. Hill's practice and then still another from the specialist. Each poses some finite risk. Whether either is worth it is a complex question. It is a question that cannot be answered based on technical considerations alone. If Ms. Forman is unusually fearful of radiation, it would be rational to take that into account in deciding the potential harms of further x-rays. She might decide to limit her exposure to the first series. On the other hand, she may be unusually unconcerned about radiation, but terribly worried about the suspicious appearance of her lung. She might rationally choose to have not only the specialist's series, but also a repeat series from her internist.

Added to the evaluation of the x-ray risk and Ms. Forman's worry about her lung are other considerations. How difficult would it be for her to travel to the specialist? Is she so happy with Dr. Hill that she would resist the referral? Who is paying for the x-ray series and how willing are they to pay for the extra series? Should she be charged for the new series?

Finally, Jean Johnson might ask whether the self-interest of the clinician is entering into the decision about recommending a repeat series and whether it ought to. Would the repeat series be of financial personal interest to either Dr. Hill or Ms. Johnson? Would a clearer picture possibly lead to keeping Ms. Forman as a patient? Would a picture of less than professional quality reflect poorly on Dr. Hill or Ms. Johnson if the original pictures are transferred to other professionals?

All these evaluations could occur to Ms. Johnson as she tries to decide what to say about repeating the series. In fact, in literally every clinical case evaluations of these kinds are going on continually. Of course, in this case and in many others, most of the evaluations may not be ethical evaluations. Some probably will be, however. For example, the decisions pertaining to the role of self-interest in recommending additional x-rays seem to verge on moral choices. Decisions about whether to respect the autonomy of the patient in deciding whether to repeat the series, especially if the radiographer or physician believes some course other than the one the patient will choose would be better for the patient, certainly raise issues of considerable moral importance. In the next case, we shall attempt to differentiate moral and nonmoral evaluations more clearly.

DISTINGUISHING MORAL FROM NONMORAL EVALUATIONS

Clearly not all evaluations that allied health personnel must make are as mundane as deciding whether additional x-rays are appropriate for a possible lung cancer patient. Some involve complex combinations of moral and nonmoral evaluations of life-saving proportions. Try to distinguish the moral and nonmoral choices in the following case involving an occupational therapist.

CASE 2: Suicidal Intentions

Mr. Smith was a 38-year-old single male with a central cord lesion being seen by Mildred Watson, an occupational therapist in a rehabilitation hospital 150 miles from his home. Mr. Smith had both upper extremity and lower extremity involvement. He had moderate upper extremity spasticity, shoulder motion, and walked with moderate assistance. The treatment goals for Mr. Smith set by occupational therapy were to improve all areas of activity of daily living functioning; improve trunk stability; measure for and adapt a wheelchair to meet all physical, personal, and functional needs; and train Mr. Smith to use the wheelchair to attain maximum independence.

Mr. Smith was seen two times daily by occupational therapy. He developed a good rapport with Ms. Watson. During one of the treatment sessions, Mr. Smith confided in her his plans to "use the wheelchair to finish the job because I do not want to live like this." Further discussion with him clarified that finishing the job meant commit suicide.

Because of the confidential nature of the conversation, Ms. Watson sought out Mr. Smith's physician prior to documenting the conversation in the patient's chart. She conveyed the specifics and tenor of the conversation to the physician. The physician, a resident on his second month of a neurology rotation, decided it was best to keep the information hushed and shared minimal information with the rest of the treatment team. The doctor appeared not to take the suicide threat seriously and directed Ms. Watson to continue treatment, avoid documenting the conversation in the chart until something more definitive had occurred, and order the wheelchair.

As treatment progressed and the delivery date for the wheelchair drew near, Ms. Watson again approached the physician about Mr. Smith's continued discussions concerning "finishing the job." The physician informed Ms. Watson that her communication was based on "speculation." Contrary to what she was saying, during the course of the physician's examinations of Mr. Smith, the patient exhibited a positive, healthy attitude concerning his disability, was satisfied with the treatment he was receiving at the Rehabilitation Center, was progressing nicely, and looked forward to getting the wheelchair and going home. The physician also noted that Mr. Smith did not exhibit any unusual moodiness and never discussed any suicidal intentions with him.

The dilemma for Ms. Watson became clear when the chair arrived. Should she ignore Mr. Smith's periodic conversations about doing himself in? Should she inform the rest of the treatment team about her conversation and ignore the physician's orders? By revealing her conversation with Mr. Smith, is she breaching patient confidentiality? Should she document the conversation in the medical record? What are the obligations placed on those responsible for the notes in the medical record? What should she do about the physician that repeatedly refused to address Mr. Smith's suicidal intention because he had no first-hand knowledge?

As with Case 1 there are many value terms in this description that signal evaluations taking place. The case mentions "treatment goals" of "improving all areas of activity, trunk stability, meeting needs, and training for maximum independence." These are all being evaluated positively. They would not be goals if they were not. The physician "thinks it is best to keep the information hushed." Ms. Watson clearly believes that suicide by the patient would be a bad thing.

Here, however, it is not as clear what kind of evaluations are taking place. When the physician says it would be best to keep the information confidential, is he saying that he thinks the outcome would be best, or is he conveying a moral judgment? Is he saying it would be morally best, perhaps because he feels there is a moral duty of confidentiality that requires nondisclosure? Likewise, in what sense does Ms. Watson believe suicide by the patient would be bad? She could be assessing the patient's overall welfare, saying that she believes that overall it would be better for the patient if he did not commit suicide. That seems like common sense, but it could be disputed. Someone could argue that, if Mr. Smith would inevitably be depressed, he might actually have his interests served by committing suicide. That, at least, is a point of view that one could imagine.

Still, Ms. Watson might respond by saying that it is simply morally wrong to fail to report the suicidal thoughts (even if the patient would be perpetually miserable while he continues to live). If she were to respond that way, she would be engaging in a *moral* evaluation.

In the introduction we distinguished between moral and nonmoral evaluations.[1] Moral evaluations are those that pertain to actions or practices or traits of character that, first, are ultimate appeals above which there is no higher standard. They are, second, universal in the sense that everyone ought, in principle, to agree with the judgment. And, third, they must not give special consideration to the good of one over another.

Ms. Watson may want to claim that failing to intervene in a potential suicide is morally wrong (even if Mr. Smith wants to end his life and would be miserable if he does not end it). According to some ethical theories, the mere fact that he would be better off dead does not make the suicide right morally. If that is Ms. Watson's claim, then she is distinguishing between moral and nonmoral senses of the right or good.

Likewise, the physician's claiming that it would be "best" to keep the conversation confidential could be saying simply that the patient would be better off if it were kept confidential (without making a moral statement at all). He could be estimating the consequences for the patient if the information were disclosed and if it were not disclosed and judging that the outcome would be better if they kept the information to themselves. He might believe that the patient is not really serious about the suicide and that disclosure would hurt the patient's reputation. He might believe that disclosure would drive the patient away from their care so that, even if he were serious about the suicide, the patient would not be helped by announcing his plan to others.

As with Ms. Watson, however, the physician may be saying it is morally best to keep the confidence. He may believe that health professionals have a moral duty to keep confidences, that they have promised to do so. He may believe that it is part of the code of their respective professions and that they each have a duty to abide by their professional codes.

The American Medical Association since 1980 has been committed to a strong pledge of confidentiality.[2] The occupational therapists' code has a similar pledge.[3] (We shall see in later cases that some of the other codes of the allied health professions have quite different requirements when it comes to the duty to keep confidences. While the codes of the physician and Ms. Watson may not be in conflict, some other allied health professionals might be forced into significant moral disagreement if they believe that their moral duty is defined by their professional group.)

This case makes clear that it will not be enough to identify when value judgments take place. They occur continually in every single case in health care, but a further distinction will have to be made to determine whether the evaluations are moral or not. Merely recognizing a value term—such as good or right or duty—will not be enough to tell whether the judgment implies morally good, morally right, or one's moral duty. Those judgments are moral only when they appeal to the highest possible standard. Whether that standard is the code of ethics of one's profession, one's religious tradition, one's society, or one's conscience will make a difference. It is to the question of what the standard should be for making moral evaluations that we now turn.

ENDNOTES

1. See the Introduction, pages xix–xxi.
2. Council on Judicial and Ethical Affairs, American Medical Association, *Current Opinions of the Council on Ethical and Judicial Affairs of the American Medical Association: Including the Principles of Medical Ethics and Rules of the Council on Ethical and Judicial Affairs* (Chicago: AMA, 1989), p. 21.
3. American Occupational Therapy Association, *Occupational Therapy Code of Ethics*, 1994.

CHAPTER 2

What Is the Source of Moral Judgments?

Once ethical and other evaluative judgments are identified in cases under consideration, the next question is: Where should one look to determine what is moral? Sometimes health professionals recognize the problem of what is moral to be a matter of "professional ethics." They might turn to the code of ethics of their profession. Allied health professionals increasingly have codes of ethics available from their professional groups. For example, for American occupational therapists this would be the current code of the American Occupational Therapy Association;[1] for medical records professionals, the *Code of Ethics* of the American Health Information Management Association.[2] There are some problems, however. First, not all occupational therapists or health information professionals may be members of their professional groups. Are the codes binding even if one is not a member? Are they binding on occupational therapists or health information professionals from other countries, for instance? It would seem odd that the American code would bind someone who is not even a member of the professional organization. Second, what should happen if two members of the health care team are from different professional groups and their codes conflict? Or even if someone is a member of a professional group, he or she might wonder whether conduct is always correct just because it conforms to the code of the professional association.

The problem could be particularly acute when an allied health professional is in disagreement with a physician over what is ethical. It seems strange that a physician would want to yield to the code of the allied health professional as an authority in such a disagreement. The physician might believe that the physician's own moral judgment or the judgment of the physician's professional group (such as the American Medical Association) is the proper standard for assessing whether the physician's prescription is morally correct. On the other hand, the allied health professional might not agree that the physician's judgment or that of his or her professional association is automatically authoritative.

An allied health professional working in a hospital may have to contend not only with the ethical code of the physician, but also with the code of the hospital. The hospital may have a locally generated code of conduct or may be subject to ethical positions taken by its sponsor or of the American Hospital Association. Should the allied health professional consider the hospital's ethical position to be the source of authority for determining what is ethical conduct?

If the hospital is sponsored by a religious organization, the hospital's ethical code may be derived from the theological ethical commitments of the religious group. For Catholic hospitals in the United States, for instance, this would be the *Ethical and Religious Directives for Catholic Health Facilities*.[3]

The allied health professional may personally stand in some religious tradition that may or may not be the same as that of the sponsoring hospital. Should a religious tradition be treated as being an authoritative source for knowing what is ethical? If so, should it be the hospital's tradition or the allied health practitioner's? And how should either of these relate to the professional code of the relevant professional associations?

Finally, the allied health practitioner will often confront ethical dilemmas involving a particular patient who also has moral standards that he or she feels should be the foundation of moral judgments involving his or her medication. Is the patient's ethical stance a defensible basis for grounding the ethical positions taken by a care giver? In this chapter, cases are presented that provide an opportunity to examine alternative ways of grounding moral judgments. In each case, the important problem upon which to focus is not so much what is the right thing to do but, rather, what is the source of moral authority and upon what authority the allied health professional's behavior should be shaped.

GROUNDING ETHICS IN THE PROFESSIONAL CODE

An allied health professional confronting an ethical problem that poses a significant difficulty may want to turn to the professional code of ethics to determine what it says regarding the issue at stake. Often the professional code will provide insight based on years of collective experience of the members of the professional group.

Sometimes the apparent answer from the code seems so appropriate that no further consideration is necessary. But in other cases it may not be obvious to the individual care giver that the profession's collective wisdom is morally definitive. One problem arises because the professional group's code can change over the years. Each time the code changes does the ethically correct behavior for the members of the profession really change or only what the professional group's members believe is the correct behavior?

What about care givers working in a field who are not members of the professional organization? Does its code determine what is ethically correct for those who are not members or only for members? Can what is ethically correct for allied health professionals change depending on whether they are members of their professional association? And what about practitioners in other nations? Does the American professional code determine what is right for them or does their own professional organization's code? It seems odd that what is right would depend on the country in which one practices and when one practices. The following case asks what the role of a professional code should be in determining what is ethically correct conduct.

CASE 3: Does the Professional Code Settle the Matter?

James Howe, a primary physician practicing in Eastern Memorial Hospital, has diagnosed Dwight Lee, a 28-year-old white male, as having acquired immune deficiency syndrome (AIDS). Mr. Lee has been referred to the Physical Therapy Department of Eastern Memorial. He is to receive hydrotherapy—whirlpool treatments—for the open skin lesions that have erupted on his buttocks. He is brought to the physical therapy by Tom Madison, a radiologic technologist who works with Dr. Howe who provides regular care for Mr. Lee.

Marilyn Edison, a physical therapist, has been assigned to provide and supervise the hydrotherapy treatment for Mr. Lee. Prior to her seeing Mr. Lee, Dr. Howe calls Ms. Edison to inform her of Mr. Lee's condition (AIDS).

During the first session that Ms. Edison has with Mr. Lee, he asks her to please keep his AIDS condition completely confidential—not to tell anyone, especially anyone in the Physical Therapy Department. It seems that Dwight Lee knows one of the staff, a physical therapy assistant in the department. Mr. Lee does not want the assistant to know that he (Lee) is gay because the assistant and he are, in Mr. Lee's words, "very close friends."

Despite the fact that "normal" protocol for hydrotherapy requires that physical therapists and physical therapy assistants wear gloves, Marilyn Edison is torn between divulging the patient's condition to the assistant and keeping the confidence. The latter seems to be consistent with the American Physical Therapy Association's ethical standards. Its code states that "Information relating to the physical therapist-patient relationship is confidential and may not be communicated to a third party not involved in that patient's care without the prior written consent of the patient, subject to applicable law." However, that code also states that "Information may be disclosed to appropriate authorities when it is necessary to protect the welfare of an individual or the community." If Ms. Edison can figure out what the code implies about disclosure to a colleague whose physical welfare may be at risk, does that settle the matter ethically?* [4]

There are obvious reasons why Marilyn Edison might want to disclose to her colleagues that Mr. Lee has AIDS. It would be a typical matter of gossip among colleagues, but that hardly seems to provide any justification for the disclosure. The diagnosis of AIDS, however, could be medically important to others working with the patient. To what extent are the other members of the health care team—physical therapists, the physician assistant, or nurses—at risk for transmission of human immunodeficiency virus (HIV) in these circumstances? Assuming that those responsible for treating and dressing the open skin lesions and giving injections are at some degree of risk (even if they use gloves and take other normal precautions), do they have an ethical right to know of the special risk in this case?

Ms. Edison cited the ethical standards of the American Physical Therapy Association as a reason why she should keep the confidence. But the standards also speak of the acceptability of disclosures necessary to protect the welfare of the patient or third parties. That raises the question of whether, for her or others, the position of the Association, if it can be discerned, is morally definitive. If she is perplexed about what is morally right, is that where she should turn? Would it be sufficient for Ms. Edison to telephone the Association and ask for clarification? Doing so seems to imply that what the Association says on an ambiguous and controversial issue is definitive.

If the professional code is the moral authority that an allied health professional should use, a problem arises. Mr. Madison, the radiologic technologist, is also an allied health professional. The code of ethics of the American Society of Radiologic Technologists in effect at the time gave a quite different opinion on the subject of confidentiality. It says that "Radiologic Technologists shall judiciously protect the patient's right to privacy and shall maintain all patient information in the strictest confidence."[5] It provides no exceptions in order to protect the welfare of third parties. This

**This case was supplied by Professor Carole Burnette, August 1989.*

could mean that it is unethical for the radiologic technologist to disclose and that simultaneously it is morally imperative for the physical therapist.

Dr. Howe may face a similar problem. The American Medical Association's *Current Opinions* specifies that for its members, "Where a patient threatens to inflict serious bodily harm to another person and there is a reasonable probability that the patient may carry out the threat, the physician should take reasonable precautions for the protection of the intended victim, including notification of law enforcement authorities."[6]

It can be debated exactly what the members of each of these groups is obligated to do in the case of a patient who poses a significant risk to members of the health care team. It could also be debated whether various members of the health care team are at a significant risk if they are not informed of the patient's HIV status. The real problem here, however, is whether each of these members of the health care team ought to treat their respective codes as definitive. If so, the physical therapist and the physician seem to have a duty that is different from the radiologic technologist. The physical therapist, according to the provision in effect at the time, should disclose whenever it will protect the welfare of the patient or community, while the radiologic technologist should not disclose no matter what. The physician should disclose only when there is a threat of serious bodily harm (not when it will protect the welfare of the patient—as is the policy of the physical therapists).

The real question raised here is whether the members of each professional group should be bound by their group's code of ethics. Is there some more definitive standard of ethics to which all three of these members of the health care team should appeal rather than simply to their own group's codes?

GROUNDING ETHICS IN THE PHYSICIAN'S ORDERS

One possible resolution in the previous case is that whenever the various allied health professional codes are in disagreement, the final authority is the judgment of the physician. In some situations a health care worker is presented with ethical decisions that seem to be grounded not so much in either public policy or professional codes but in the beliefs of practicing physicians. Of course, the physician, in reaching his or her moral conclusion, may have to decide how important the physician's professional code is, but by the time the physician has decided on a course of action, the allied health professional may be presented only with the "doctor's order." The following two cases raise the question of whether allied health professionals should treat the moral judgments incorporated into a physician's instruction as definitive for their own work.

CASE 4: Disagreeing with the Physician's Moral Judgment

Bessy Whitney is an 87-year-old woman who has incurable cancer. She came into the hospital two days ago. At the time of Mrs. Whitney's admission, Jerry Stephens, a respiratory care practitioner, was in the room when Mrs. Whitney said to the physician who admitted her that she did not want any heroics. She made it clear that this meant no ventilators.

On the second day of her hospitalization, Mrs. Whitney has a medical crisis. Mr. Stephens is summoned to Mrs. Whitney's room where the nurse indicates that the admitting physician has ordered ventilation for Mrs. Whitney. When Mr. Stephens hears this order, he questions it because he was there when Mrs. Whitney said that she didn't want any heroics. The nurse is upset, but says that the physician had decided that even though she had refused the ventilation, he had decided that it was in her best interest to get it.

At the time of this confrontation, the physician cannot be reached. What should Mr. Stephens do?

The physician in this case seems to have made a moral decision that it is his duty to do what he thinks will be in the patient's best interest even when she has refused the treatment. That is an approach that was quite common among physicians in the past. The Hippocratic Oath bound physicians to do what they thought would benefit their patients. Many physicians interpreted this to mean that they should do anything that would preserve life. It was the decision made by Karen Quinlan's physician.[7] Today it seems clear that physicians are much more likely to respect the wishes of patients in such cases, but some physicians still believe that morally they are permitted (or required) to do what they think is best in these situations, even if it means overriding the patient's wishes.

This physician has apparently reached this moral conclusion. The American Medical Association's *Current Opinions* affirms that the preference of the individual patient should prevail when he or she is terminally ill, but "Unless it is clearly established that the patient is terminally ill or permanently unconscious, a physician should not be deterred from appropriately aggressive treatment of a patient."[8] If he believed this patient was not actually terminally ill, then his position would be consistent with his profession's code. Perhaps the physician's views are shaped by his interpretation of his professional code or perhaps he has reached his conclusion on some other basis. It should be clear that nothing technical in medical science is at stake. The issue is whether, on the basis of the physician's instruction, it is morally right to prolong her life through the use of the ventilator when she has expressed a wish not to have it used.

The issue facing Mr. Stephens is whether the physician's judgment is definitive here. There are both legal and ethical considerations. Legally, Mrs. Whitney is being treated without her consent. If Mr. Stephens provides the treatment, he is a party to the illegal act.

But there is also a moral issue here. Possibly it is moral to ventilate even if it turns out to be illegal. Should Mr. Stephens view the moral judgment of the physician as definitive? Is it any more definitive than the various professional codes to which the nurse and respiratory care practitioner might turn or is the physician's personal moral judgment unimportant in helping Mr. Stephens decide what he ought to do? The following case raises a similar issue.

CASE 5: Disputing a Physician's Clinical Judgment

In July, 1989, a 27-year-old female was admitted to the city general hospital. She was diagnosed as drug addicted. She had elevated blood pressure, renal insufficiency, and end-stage renal disease (ESRD). Doctors had hoped that they could avoid dialysis through controlling her problems with medication and diet.

Diet instruction was ordered. She was placed on a renal diet. The dietitian planned to provide information for a patient in ESRD (very restricted diet, that is, low protein, low potassium, and low sodium). But one of the residents (doctors) asked the dietitian to give only information on protein (that is, the level of protein the patient should have) and a list of foods with the protein level of each. According to nutritional reference books and the diet manual, the patient should restrict potassium and possibly fluid instead of only protein and sodium. What should the dietitian do?

This case at first looks much like the first case. In both the allied health professional disagrees with the action of the physician. In Case 4, however, the disagreement was clearly moral. Both respiratory care practitioner and physician understood the patient was dying and did not want to be ventilated. The physician, however, believed that morally his duty was to preserve life even if the patient disagreed. In this case, it is less obvious what the basis of the disagreement is. Possibly the resident realized that standard procedure included paying attention to potassium, sodium, and fluids as well as protein. He might have made the decision that that was not worth doing because it was too expensive or too time consuming. If asked, he might have said something like, "An addict isn't worth it." Then the dietitian's dilemma would have been what standard to use in disagreeing with these moral judgments of the resident. The problem would be similar to the previous case. The dietitian would have to decide whether the moral judgments of this resident were definitive for her.

Quite possibly, however, the dispute is not moral at all. They may simply have different understandings of what is clinically important for this patient. If the dispute is over the (nonmoral) judgments about the usefulness of restricting potassium, then the dietitian's problem is quite different. She needs to decide whether the physician's clinical judgment (not his moral judgment) is authoritative. While in medical matters we often think of the physician as the "captain of the health care team," it seems obvious that, on occasion, they can err. In fact, on a question of dietary restrictions for patients in end-stage renal failure, the dietitian may well know more than the physician. Now the problem is no longer what the source of moral authority is. It is what the allied health professional should do when a technical error seems to have been made. What options are open to the dietitian?

GROUNDING ETHICS IN HOSPITAL POLICY

If the allied health professional cannot automatically ground ethical judgments in the physician's moral views or professional codes specifying what professionals believe is ethically correct, can the institution in which a health care provider works provide that grounding? Many allied health professionals work in hospitals or other health care institutions that have codes of ethics of their own. They may be in hospitals sponsored by large organizations—public or private—that have ethical standards, or they may be in a local institution that, through its board of trustees or its medical board, has formally adopted a statement or code of conduct about what is believed to be ethical. To what extent should the allied health professional working within these institutions feel bound by such statements? To what extent is the institution the "source" of the health care provider's ethical obligation?

CASE 6: Is Hospital Policy Moral?

While performing a routine review of the record of a currently hospitalized patient at an inpatient mental health facility, Mary Kantian, the health information administrator, notes an entry by a staff occupational therapist that she had seen a visitor selling drugs to this and two other patients on the unit.

Although this is documented in the patient record, hospital policy also calls for filing of an incident report in such an instance; the incident report would ordinarily initiate an investigation and appropriate corrective action. There is no indication that an incident report has been filed, and when the health information administrator asks the occupational therapist (OT) about this, the OT states that she has not done so because of fear of potential reprisals by the drug dealer, either against her or against the three patients who are the dealer's customers.

If one followed the traditional ethics of the health care professions here, the obligation of the occupational therapist and the health information administrator would be to follow the course of action that would benefit the patient. Mary Kantian or the occupational therapist might have concluded that it was in the interests of her patients to insist that the report be filed (in order to try to eliminate the risk of continued drug use). On the other hand, they might have concluded, as apparently the occupational therapist did, that the risk of reprisals made it contrary to the interests of her patients to file the report.

The case is made more complicated by the fact that the occupational therapist also claimed that it was contrary to her own interests to file the report. While traditional health care ethics that focus exclusively on the welfare of the patient would consider the provider's interests irrelevant, other ethical principles (such as classical utilitarian ethics) would include all envisioned benefits and harms (including those of the provider herself).

This case is made still more complex by the fact that there is a clearly understood hospital policy requiring the filing of incident reports in such cases. Presumably, the administrators in adopting this policy have considered the case when it is contrary to the patient's or the provider's interests to file reports and have adopted a rule nonetheless requiring that the report be filed.

Now the problem is: What weight should be given to the fact that writers of the hospital policy have adopted a position, arguably a moral position, that requires reporting in such situations? By agreeing to work in the institution have the occupational therapist and the health information administrator acknowledged that the hospital authorities are morally definitive (at least for matters arising in the course of carrying out hospital duties)? Should the hospital's policy be treated as the definitive standard for such moral judgments? If not, how much weight should it be given and what other sources should the occupational therapist and the medical records administrator turn to in order to decide what is moral in this situation? The next case pits the judgments of the physician, the professional code, and the hospital against another possible source of ethical obligation: the patient's ethical judgments.

GROUNDING ETHICS IN THE PATIENT'S VALUES

Another possibility for the source of the ethical and other evaluations that necessarily are incorporated into the health care worker's decisions is the patient. It is sometimes believed that, since there are so many different ethical positions possible on controversial issues, every person should have the right to choose his or her own ethics (or at least should have the right to act as if his or her position were the right one). A slightly different view, referred to by philosophers as *personal relativism*, is that to say something is ethical literally means nothing more than that it is the position approved by the speaker. According to this view, if one believes that an action is morally right, it literally is right; that is the final standard. On the other hand, someone else may have a quite different perspective. For the other person, the same action could, for him or her, be wrong. There is no further appeal beyond the individual.[9] The following case poses the problem of whether the health care provider should treat the patient as the source of moral standards.

CASE 7: Is the Patient Always Right?

A 38-year-old woman was admitted through the emergency room to the hospital after having taken 50 Seconal tablets. On discharge, the face sheet of the patient record was incomplete; no final diagnosis was recorded. The coder in the Medical Records Department reviewed the record and noted that, in addition to the Emergency Room notes, the nurses' notes described measures that were instituted against suicide and a physician reference on the discharge summary that the "patient no longer demonstrated suicidal tendencies..."

Based on this, the coder assigned the following diagnostic codes to be used for billing purposes as well as for diagnostic indices that are maintained for research and educational purposes.

967.0 Poisoning by barbiturates

E950.1 Suicide (attempted) and self-inflicted poisoning by barbiturates

Approximately three weeks after discharge, the patient accounts manager was contacted by the patient, who was very upset that the insurance company had denied payment of the hospitalization because the policy did not cover hospitalizations resulting from suicide attempt. She was outraged with her insurer because they had repeatedly denied her payment for needed psychiatric care. She insisted that she had become suicidal because of the insurance company's unfair treatment and that they at least owed her coverage for the emergency. She indicated that if the only way to get them to pay for the emergency room care was to call the episode an accident, then ethically that was the right thing to do.

The patient accounts manager discussed the situation with the director of the Medical Records Department, who reviewed the available data and contacted the attending physician. The physician indicated that he had not stated the diagnosis as a suicide gesture, but that he also did not dispute the accuracy of the coding. This information was reviewed with the patient accounts manager, who referred the situation to the hospital administrator. Shortly thereafter, the director of the Medical Records Department received instructions from the administrator to change the diagnostic codes to accidental poisoning for resubmission to the insurance company for payment of the bill.

The medical records administrator, according to the opinion of her professional organization, has a moral duty to "refuse to perform or conceal acts that are fraudulent, questionable or unprofessional."[10] On the other hand, the administrator of the hospital has apparently reviewed the situation and determined that the patient has a case.

The medical records administrator has several forces impinging on her claiming some kind of moral authority including the hospital policy as articulated by the administrator, the *Code of Ethics* of the American Health Information Management Association (AHIMA), and moral claims of the patient. Increasingly, the patient's rights movement is insisting that patients are their own moral authorities and that they have the right to determine on their own whether an act is right or wrong from them. What is the relative significance of these different moral standards for this medical records administrator? How should they have a bearing on her own sense of what is morally right and wrong as determined by her own moral reflection, her religious and philosophical convictions, and her own conscience? The following case forces us to examine the role of religious and philosophical convictions and personal conscience in relation to these other sources of moral authority.

GROUNDING ETHICS IN RELIGIOUS OR PHILOSOPHICAL PERSPECTIVES

Allied health professionals sometimes will find that they or the people with whom they are interacting claim they are not grounding their ethical positions in professional codes, the opinions of physicians, hospitals, or patients, but see them as coming from certain religious or philosophical perspectives. The problem can be especially acute when, as in the following case, the health care provider senses that his or her own religious or philosophical perspective may conflict with the professional code.

CASE 8: Religious Objections to Working on the Abortion Service

Sandra Goldberg is a lab technician in the Obstetrics Department of City Hospital in a conservative state. They had never performed abortions until a recent hospital board of trustees decision that reluctantly affirmed that, since abortions were legal, and the hospital was a state institution, they ought to do their share. They were concerned that too many women in the community were leaving the area to obtain expensive abortions in a distant state. Poor women were simply not getting services or were resorting to nonprofessional attempts to abort their unwanted pregnancies.

No one in the hospital was happy about this decision. The hospital made every effort to permit physicians and nurses who conscientiously objected to abortions to be relieved of any obligation to perform them. As sometimes happens, the broad policy debate at the level of the hospital administration did not specifically address the responsibilities of other members of the health care team who might have to be involved.

Ms. Goldberg was one who would be affected. She was responsible for all lab work on her shift for patients scheduled for obstetrical surgery. She was also an Orthodox Jew. She had accepted the rabbinical interpretation that abortion is morally prohibited and wondered whether she could in any way participate in the abortion procedure by doing the lab work associated with it. In contrast to the physicians and nurses, there was no easy way that she could divert the work to a colleague.

She was aware that not all Jews objected to abortion. She was also aware that the code of ethics of the laboratory technicians' association did not oppose abortion and, in fact, states that clinical laboratory professionals have as their "primary objective to ensure a high standard of care for the patients they serve."[11] The physician who is chairman of obstetrics and the hospital policy reluctantly supports the right of persons to obtain an abortion and has concluded that hospital personnel ought to do their fair share in providing the service. Ms. Goldberg's professional code poses no objection and no clear basis for her to object to participating. Her rabbi insists that her participation is immoral. What role should each of these have in shaping her moral conscience?*

This case finally gets to the crux of the question of how individual moral conscience should be shaped. Ms. Goldberg is subjected to claims for moral authority that are similar to those confronted in previous cases in this chapter: professional codes, physician judgment, hospital policy, and patient opinion. In addition, Ms. Goldberg confronts a claim from her religious tradition that it can determine what is ethical conduct.

How should Ms. Goldberg respond in the light of these claims? We have seen that there is some reason to doubt that a behavior is morally right simply because a professional code, a physician, a hospital, or a patient says so. Is Ms. Goldberg, then, free, in the light of this simply to form her own conscience using her own considered opinion as the ultimate standard?

Some people may believe that there is no more ultimate appeal beyond their considered judgments. Ms. Goldberg, however, is, by her own admission, a member of a community that claims to have a way of knowing what is morally right. Presumably, joining such a community (or deciding to remain in it) conveys at least a general acceptance of the claims of the group that it has a way of knowing about moral matters.

**This case was supplied by Dr. Glinda Price.*

Thus, part of being a Roman Catholic is to accept certain beliefs about the authority of the Pope and Church councils, about the authority of scripture and tradition. Part of being a Protestant is to accept the claim that only the Bible is a definitive source of religious knowledge (including knowledge of religious ethics). Accepting (at least to some degree) these beliefs about how one knows what is moral is part of the essence of claiming to be an adherent to one of these traditions. It would be logically inconsistent to say "I am a Catholic in good standing, yet I totally reject that the Church's views are relevant on the question of how we know what is moral." One could argue that Ms. Goldberg's acknowledgment that she is a member of a certain religious community is simultaneously an acknowledgment that, for her, Jewish ways of knowing what is morally required are definitive or ultimate.

It seems that being a member of any of the other organizations is a quite different matter. For Ms. Goldberg to join the American Society for Medical Technology does not seem to imply or require that one assume that the group is authoritative in moral matters. Likewise, to join the health care team at City Hospital does not seem to imply that the hospital's administration has definitive moral authority. Ms. Goldberg's problem, while she forms her conscience, is to determine which, if any, of these individuals and groups exerting moral claims on her really have any claim to her attention. If you were Ms. Goldberg, which, if any, would you consider authoritative?

ENDNOTES

1. American Occupational Therapy Association, *Occupational Therapy Code of Ethics,* 1994.
2. American Health Information Management Association, *Code of Ethics* (Chicago, IL: AHIMA, amended October 1991).
3. United States Catholic Conference, Department of Health Affairs, *Ethical and Religious Directives for Catholic Health Facilities* (Washington, DC: USCC, 1975).
4. American Physical Therapy Association, *Guide for Professional Conduct,* July, 1994.
5. American Society of Radiologic Technologists, "Principle 5," in *Code of Ethics* (Albuquerque, NM: ASRT, revised March 1990). This provision has now been changed to permit breaking of confidences to protect third parties.
6. American Medical Association (AMA), Judicial Council, *Current Opinions of the Council on Ethical and Judicial Affairs of the American Medical Association—1986: Including the Principles of Medical Ethics and Rules of the Council on Ethical and Judicial Affairs* (Chicago: AMA, 1989), p. 21.
7. *In re Quinlan,* 70 N.J. 10, 355 A. 2d 647 (1976), *cert. denied* sub nom.; *Garger*

v. *New Jersey,* 429 U.S. 922 (1976), overruled in part; *In re Conroy,* 98 N.J. 321, 486 A.2d 1209 (1985).

8. AMA, *Current Opinions of the Council on Ethical and Judicial Affairs of the American Medical Association,* p. 13.
9. For a discussion of the notion of relativism in ethics see Richard B. Brandt, *Ethical Theory: The Problems of Normative and Critical Ethics* (Englewood Cliffs, NJ: Prentice Hall, 1959), pp. 271-294.
10. American Health Information Management Association, *Code of Ethics.*
11. American Society for Medical Technology, "Principle II," in *Code of Ethics* (Washington, DC: ASMT, n.d.)

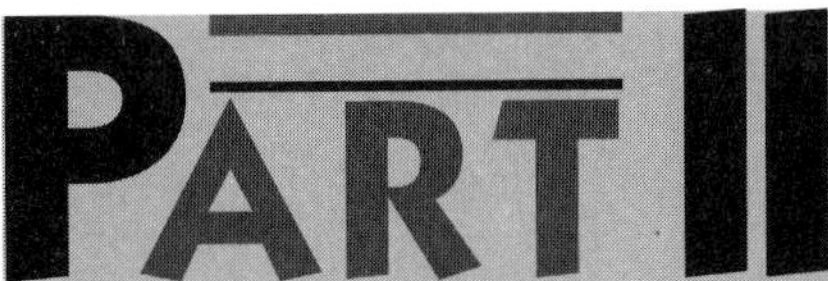

ETHICS AND VALUES IN ALLIED HEALTH

CHAPTER 3

Benefiting the Client and Others

THE DUTY TO DO GOOD AND AVOID HARM

One way to approach ethical decision making in allied health is to examine principles that describe general characteristics of actions that tend to make them morally right. In the introduction the principles of beneficence (doing good), nonmaleficence (avoiding harm), fidelity, autonomy, veracity, avoidance of killing, and justice were mentioned. From the perspective taken in Part II of this book, ethical problems in health care and elsewhere can be viewed as involving conflicts among these principles. In other cases the moral problem arises over the interpretation of one of these principles.

The idea that it is ethically right to do good, especially good for the patient, is one of the most obvious in health care ethics. The Hippocratic Oath has the health care professional pledge to "benefit the patient according to [the health care provider's] ability and judgment." The various codes of ethics of the health professions emphasize benefiting the patient or promoting the patient's welfare. The American Occupational Therapy Association code begins with the statement that occupational therapy personnel shall demonstrate a concern for the well-being of the recipient of their services. It refers to this as the principle of "beneficence."[1] The American Speech-Language-Hearing Association *Code of Ethics* begins, "Individuals shall hold paramount the welfare of persons served professionally."[2] The *Code of Ethics* of the Physician Assistant Profession expands this commitment so that physician assistants are committed to "assuming as their primary responsibility the health, safety, welfare and dignity of all humans."[3] These are all examples of what is often called the "principle of beneficence," the idea that actions or practices are morally right insofar as they produce good (for the patient or for others). The Hippocratic version, what can be called "Hippocratic beneficence," holds that an action or practice is right insofar as it produces good for (or promotes the welfare of) the patient. The first two of these codes are examples of Hippocratic beneficence; the third extends beneficence to "all humans" and might be referred to as the principle of "general beneficence" or "social beneficence."

While it seems so obvious that actions are right when they produce good that it might seem like a platitude, in fact, many serious moral problems arise over the interpretation of this principle.

First, even if it is agreed the benefits and harms that ought to be the focus of the health care professional's concern should be the patient's, there is still considerable room for controversy. The first group of cases in this chapter provides an opportunity to sort out exactly what it means to benefit the patient and protect the patient from harm.

Equally controversial is the question of whether the health care worker should limit his or her concern to benefits and harms that accrue to the patient alone as the occupational therapy code suggests or should expand the horizon to others in society as well, as suggested by the physician assistants. For example, what if protecting the patient will come at considerable risk of harm to society in general or to specific identifiable people who are not patients? What if the interests of the profession conflict with those of the patient? Or what if doing what is necessary to help the patient conflicts with the interests of the health care professional's family? Is it obvious that the health care provider should place the patient's interest above those of the professional's own family? These are the problems of the cases in the second section of this chapter.

BENEFITING THE PATIENT

Assume for the time being that it is agreed that an important moral principle is that the health care provider should act so as to benefit the patient or client—as the *Occupational Therapy Code of Ethics* says, "demonstrate concern for the well-being of the recipient of . . . services." Even limiting our concern to this apparently simple principle turns out to raise serious problems of interpretation. For example, many ethical systems, such as the occupational therapists' code, take as their goal producing good or welfare in general. They do not limit the benefits to health and safety. Other health care ethics state that the moral duty of the health professional is to promote the health of the patient. The first case in this section forces the allied health professional to decide what should happen when nonhealth benefits might outweigh the health risks. Later cases examine the relation, first, between producing good and avoiding harm for the patient and, second, between determining the good produced by various rules and that produced by considering individual cases.

1. Health in Conflict with Other Goods

Health professionals are normally committed to restoring, maintaining, or improving the health of patients. Health is viewed by virtually ·ryone as a good, as something intrinsically desirable. Yet there are other goods that rational people desire as well. These include and discontent with the prescribed regimen leads them to abandon temporarily his medical goals in favor of his immediate emotional and social well-being. They may feel that his overall interests are served by some compromise with his medical interests. Other than a simple misunderstanding requiring further attempts at education, what other reason could be given for the Martins' behavior?

Assuming some account such as this, Ms. Karticoff's dilemma is one of how occupational therapy goals should be related to broader goals of Mark's happiness and the family's harmonious interaction. Should Ms. Karticoff strive to pursue Mark's well-being focusing solely on the orthopedic-neuromuscular and other medical interests or should she take a broader perspective including Mark's overall happiness and the smooth, harmonious functioning of the family?

One problem that will have to be addressed later is whether the parents' judgments about their child's overall well-being should necessarily be taken as the best possible estimate of his interests. Possibly Ms. Karticoff and the Martins have different estimates of what will provide Mark's overall well-being. Should the Martins' estimate be taken as the guiding one and why? Ms. Karticoff is a dedicated health professional. She has chosen to spend her life in occupational therapy. Could it be that she is overemphasizing the importance of the orthopedic-neuromuscular element in Mark's well-being at the expense of other elements? On the other hand, should the parents' estimate of Mark's well-being always rule? More on this issue will arise in the cases of Chapter 13, when we deal with issues of consent and the right to refuse treatment.

2. Relating Benefits and Harms

After the problem of relating health benefits to overall benefits is solved, a second question needs to be addressed if the allied health professional is to figure out what it means to do what will benefit the patient. Often the intervention that offers the greatest prospect for benefit is also more risky; it offers not only the greatest good, but also the greatest risk for harm. How is the health care provider to relate the benefits and harms in attempting to determine what will produce the most benefit?

One possibility is to approach the problem arithmetically. The benefits could be viewed as "pluses" and the harms as "minuses" on a common scale. According to this view the harms are subtracted from the goods to determine what course will do the most "net" good. This is the position of many utilitarian philosophers. It is sometimes identified with the great nineteenth-century British utilitarian Jeremy Bentham.[5] In carrying out such mental calculations, one has to factor in the probability of each envisioned benefit or harm. Some of these benefits and harms are rather easily quantifiable, such as expected numbers of years of life added with an intervention. Others, such as pain and suffering or the benefit of getting to see a loved one can, at best, be approximated. Policy analysts have developed sophisticated strategies for estimating such benefits and harms. For example, the quality-adjusted life year (QALY) is designed to take into account not only the number of years of life, but also the quality of the years.[6]

It is not obvious morally that it is correct to pursue the course of action that is expected to produce the greatest net good. Many believe there are moral constraints on such action based on other moral principles, principles to be explored in cases in later chapters. But even for those who limit their ethics to beneficence (doing good) and nonmaleficence (avoiding evil), there are problems. For example, one might try to maximize the benefit-harm ratio rather than maximize the net good calculated by subtracting the expected harm from the expected benefits. This approaches the problem of relating benefits and harms geometrically rather than arithmetically. If one imagines two courses, the second of which has twice the expected benefit and twice the expected harm, according to the ratios method there is no difference between the two, but according to the method of subtracting harms from benefits, one is always obliged to choose the high-gain/high-risk option since the difference between the expected benefit and expected harm will be greater.

Still another way of relating benefits to harms is to give nonmaleficence, the duty to avoid harming, a moral priority over beneficence. According to this view, the duty to not harm is more compelling than the duty to help. One is morally free to try to help only when one is sure that harm will not be done. In contrast to the approach that calculates net good done, giving priority to avoiding harm gives a preference to the more cautious course. In fact, if carried to an extreme, it would always lead to doing nothing. In that case, at least one would have avoided harming (even though one would also have missed opportunities to do good). The following case provides an opportunity to compare different ways of comparing benefits and harms of alternative courses of action.

CASE 10: The Conflict Between Producing Benefits and Avoiding Harms

Mrs. Julia White has been a quadriplegic for more than five years. Despite the fact that she is in an environment where there is sufficient assistance to help her stand approximately one hour per day, she refuses to do so. Standing has been shown to be effective in reducing gallstones and osteoporosis.

Ed Mills, a physical therapist, has been working with a home health care agency for six months. During this period, Mr. Mills has been seeing Mrs. White twice per week for therapy.

Despite Mr. Mills' urging, Mrs. White refuses to stand the prescribed amount of time. She refuses to stand because she says, "It is too darn uncomfortable to stand, and, besides, I don't see any difference." She hasn't developed gallstones, and there is no visible evidence of osteoporosis. Furthermore, she says, "I am terrified that I might fall." Once, two years prior, she had fallen or been dropped when she was being assisted to stand by a family member.

Mr. Mills realizes that there are both potential benefits and risks of harm if he encourages Mrs. White to stand. Sometimes he has heard that the health provider's ethical duty is to avoid causing harm to patients. The slogan is *primum non nocere*, "first of all, do no harm." He thinks that gives him a special moral obligation to avoid risking injury to his patients. Other times he hears that the duty of the therapist is to do what is best for the patient, where what is best takes into account both benefits and harms. Should he pursue a plan of encouraging Mrs. White to stand?*

This case poses several problems in deciding how to benefit the patient. First, the problem confronted in the previous case arises here as well. Mrs. White may not really be interested in maximizing her *medical* well-being; she may be interested in her total welfare, taking into account the discomfort and other psychological burdens of making the effort to stand. Mr. Mills may be focusing more narrowly on her medical welfare: the gallstones and osteoporosis. Is Mr. Mills' proper concern the health of Mrs. White measured narrowly, or should he be willing to sacrifice her medical welfare for other, broader aspects?

Once that question is resolved, there remains the question of how Mr. Mills should relate benefits and harms. If he were a straight utilitarian, he would envision all the benefits of encouraging his patient to stand and then envision all the harms. He would then estimate the probabilities of those benefits and harms and multiply by those probabilities to get the estimated quantity of benefit and harm. Finally, he would subtract the harms from the benefits to get a net amount of good for his patient. His moral duty would be to get that net number of positives minus negatives as large as possible (even if that meant risking a great deal of harm, provided the projected good offset the harm and left the largest possible net of expected good).

**This case was provided by Professor Carole Burnette.*

There are other things he could do with these estimates of benefit and harm, however. He could calculate the ratio of benefits to harms and strive for the largest possible ratio. Would that produce the same result as subtracting the benefits from the harms in this case?

There is a third possibility, suggested by the slogan, "first of all, do no harm." He could say that his first priority morally is to make sure that he minimizes the harm that he does to Mrs. White. Even if great good could come from aggressively intervening (pushing hard to get her standing), he could consider it morally more important that he not add to her misery and cause her new harms. He could insist on avoiding harm even if avoiding the possible harm also prevented a chance to help. Which of the strategies for relating benefits and harms is the most conservative? Which is the most interventionist? How should Mr. Mills relate the benefits and harms in this case?

3. Benefits of Rules and Benefits in Specific Cases

Even if the health care provider solves the problem of relating benefits to harms as well as the problem of relating health to nonhealth benefits, there is still another difficulty in figuring out what will benefit the patient. Some people who calculate consequences do so with reference to the specific case considered in isolation. They look only at the effects of alternative actions in the specific case. Others are equally focused on consequences, but they are interested in the consequences of alternative rules. Those people, who were referred to as "rule utilitarians" in the introduction, hold that one should look at the consequences of alternative rules and choose the rule that produces consequences as good or better than any alternative. Then, once the rule is adopted, morality requires that it be followed without reassessment in specific cases. Only at the stage of adopting rules do consequences count according to this view. Holders of this view oppose case-by-case calculations either for pragmatic reasons—because they think there is too much room for error in the heat of a crisis—or for theoretical reasons—because morality is simply a matter of playing by the rules once they have been adopted.[7] The following case illustrates how these two approaches to calculating consequences impact on a health professional's moral choices.

CASE 11: A Dying Patient on a Low-Salt Diet

Mr. Millard Jasper is a 77-year-old man diagnosed as having a metastatic carcinoma of the prostate. He had been hospitalized many times for surgery and other procedures. He has now returned to the hospital for what appears to be the last time. Both the patient and the health care team know the end is near. They expect that he has at most two to three weeks to live. He is being kept comfortable with IV morphine, but his condition continues to decline.

Mary Masterson was the dietitian at Hebron General Hospital where Mr. Jasper is hospitalized. She was surprised to see that his oncologist had ordered a low-salt diet for Mr. Jasper. Ms. Masterson realized that Mr. Jasper had a history of high blood pressure. She concurred that normally a low-salt diet was appropriate for such patients, but she considered this case to be different.

Mr. Jasper had protested loudly on previous occasions when his diet was restricted. He had complained that life wasn't worth living if he couldn't taste his food. Now Ms. Masterson could not imagine what the reasoning was for the oncologist's order for the low-salt diet. She thought to herself that there was almost no chance that salt could harm Mr. Jasper at this point. In fact, the thought crossed her mind that a cardiac event that shortened Mr. Jasper's life at this point might even be a blessing. Ms. Masterson had often complained about the foolishness of special diets to prevent long-term problems in terminally ill patients.

She asked the oncologist about the order, believing that he probably would change it, but she was mistaken. He gruffly muttered that he had his reasons, and when he orders a low-salt diet, it is a low-salt diet he wants.

Ms. Masterson was sure he really did not have a reason. Based on her conversations with Mr. Jasper, she was sure the patient had not and would not consent to the low-salt order if he understood it. Still, she knew that the standard practice was for the dietitian to provide the diet as prescribed. She had shown the courage to question the order, but now the oncologist was making clear that he was insisting on the limit on the diet. She also knew that she could provide the salt for Mr. Jasper and that the oncologist would never know the difference. She was absolutely sure it would be better for the patient, all things considered, if she bent the rule and circumvented the physician's order. At the same time she knew that such rules had their purpose. She wondered whether the hospital would be a better place if all members of the health care team circumvented physician orders when they believed the patient would be better off. At the same time she was really convinced she had calculated Mr. Jasper's interests correctly this time. Should she slip the salt onto the tray?

This is a classical case of the tension between the wisdom of following the rules and making an exception when one is sure that the rule doesn't work in the particular case. Ms. Masterson surely understood the function of rules in such cases, but also was very confident that this was a case when the patient's interests would be served by breaking the rule requiring members of the health care team to follow the physician's orders.

If one were a *situational utilitarian,* then the right thing to do would be to calculate the likely outcomes in the specific case with various alternative courses of action. She should imagine the benefits and harms of providing the salt and those of following the order not to provide it. She should then follow the course of action that is expected to produce the most good. While a classical social utilitarian would consider the benefits and harms for all parties—the dietitian as well as the patient—a traditional Hippocratic consequentialist will focus only on the benefits and harms for the patient. If Ms. Masterson is a situational Hippocratic consequentialist, she will provide the salt if she is convinced that it will lead to more good for her patient.

She need not ignore the rules entirely. Situationalists are willing to let rules serve as guidelines or rules of thumb. She would realize that the general rule of members of the team following physician orders usually produces more good for the patient than a policy in which each member of the team independently calculated consequences and acted accordingly. Still, for the situationalist the rules are only guidelines. It is assumed there will be special cases in which the rules don't lead to the best results, and in those cases the rules should be broken.

If Ms. Masterson holds to the *rules-of-practice* view, she will give the rule to follow the physician's orders more weight. She will assess the rule by the overall consequences of the rule comparing those consequences to those of alternative rules. Here she may ask, "What would happen if all my colleagues on the health care team used their own judgment?" She may conclude that the risk of erroneous calculations, conflicting actions by team members, and overall harm is greater if individuals use their own judgment than if they follow the rules. They may hold that once the rule is in place, it should not be violated lightly. This does not necessarily mean it can never be broken, but it should not give way just because the consequences appear to be better if the rule is ignored. Exceptions would be reserved for only the most extreme, special cases.

BENEFITING SOCIETY AND THOSE WHO ARE NOT PATIENTS

The focus of benefit in the cases thus far in this chapter is the patient. Occasionally, benefits to others emerged in the cases, but it was usually in a very marginal way. In other situations the health care provider appears caught between doing what will benefit the patient and doing something else that will have much greater benefit for other parties.

According to the classical Hippocratic ethic, the health professional was, in such cases, to choose to benefit the patient. The code of the American Occupational Therapy Association seems to follow the same pattern committing the therapist to the "well-being of the recipient of their services,"[8] while, as we have seen, the physician assistants' code commits to the welfare and dignity of "all humans."[9]

As early as the nineteenth century the codes began to realize that sometimes the moral obligation of the health professional extended beyond the individual patient. The emergence of public health in the nineteenth century suggested that sometimes the health professional had to consider the welfare of the population as a whole. More recently, health professionals have recognized ethical tensions created by their obligation to others such as the family of patients, the profession as a whole, or their own families. These cases raise this conflict between benefits to the patient and to others.

1. Benefits to Society

During the past century health professionals have gradually reached the conclusion that they bear responsibilities not only to individual patients but also to the community or to groups of people. Many codes of the health professions have incorporated similar notions of the professional's duty to the community (as opposed to the individual patient).

The ethically difficult issue is what should happen when the allied health professional's opportunity to serve the public comes at the expense of the individual patient. Health care providers are variously asked to participate in medical research for the purpose of creating generalizable knowledge, in public health campaigns, and in cost-containment efforts. None of these is ethically possible on strictly Hippocratic (individual patient welfare) grounds. The next two cases force an allied health professional to choose between serving the community (or groups of nonpatients) and serving an individual patient.

CASE 12: Helping a Patient Cheat

Sue Watkins, a physical therapist at the Hoffman Rehabilitation Clinic, overheard Janet Cook, a colleague therapist, while Ms. Cook was providing whirlpool therapy for Jim Holst. Mr. Holst, a warehouse laborer, had injured his hip in a fall four weeks earlier.

Mr. Holst had been receiving full pay during the time when he was unable to work. He made clear to Ms. Cook that he liked the idea of being paid without working. He was interested in making it appear that his injury remained so severe that he could not return to work.

At this point Ms. Watkins heard Ms. Cook explain in detail to Mr. Holst how to hold his leg when it was being manipulated by the orthopedist and how to describe the pain if he wanted to continue to be certified as unable to work.

Ms. Cook is a salaried employee of the clinic. She will get no direct financial reward for continuing the therapy. In fact, she will probably end up having to provide additional therapy. She feels she has a duty as a clinical professional to take into account only the welfare of the patient. She is convinced that Mr. Holst would be better off knowing how to describe his pain and feign the continued injury.

It seems plausible that, if the physical therapist's only moral duty is to do what will benefit the patient, then Ms. Cook has a good case for helping Mr. Holst get the maximum therapy. It might be argued that lying about the pain is unethical, but, in this case, it really would seem to help the patient.

What is Ms. Cook's obligation, if any, to the employer and the other workers whose lives will be burdened and whose health insurance program will be depleted? Should the fellow workers be considered as "patients" whose interests also need to be taken into account? Should their interests be taken into account even if they are not considered patients?

Is Mr. Holst a patient of Ms. Watkins? If not, then is her duty in this situation different from that of Ms. Cook? In calculating the benefits and harms in this case, it seems obvious that Ms. Cook could do more good overall spending her time helping someone else. It would leave more funds available for the employees to use for other purposes that must be more valuable than the benefits Mr. Holst would get. Are these physical therapists obligated to maximize the total amount of good they can do (the utilitarian option) or are the obligated to maximize the good for the patient (the Hippocratic option).

CASE 13: Providing Marginal Therapy

Shirley Dennelsten, an occupational therapist, is working for a private agency. Elmer Lantress, a 64-year-old man who has had a cerebral vascular accident (CVA), has been referred for services. The OT's employer says the patient should receive two one-half hour treatments per day. After evaluating the patient the OT tells her boss that the patient needs only one treatment per day. The employer tells the OT to do as she wishes regarding the number of daily treatments provided but that she must document two daily treatments because that is what is allowed by the third-party payor.*

As in the previous case, it seems clear that Mr. Lantress would be better off with the treatment than without it. Admittedly, he does not "need" the treatment, but it is not likely to hurt and may actually benefit him some. If Ms. Dennelsten really has as her only moral duty service to the interests of the patient, it seems clear that she should provide the two sessions per day. Her employer is, according to this view, part way right. Of course, the employer seems more interested in how many sessions are billed than how many are delivered, but, even based on what the self-serving employer has said, Ms. Dennelsten would be within her rights to provide the maximally benefiting two sessions per day.

What would be the basis of Ms. Dennelsten's objection? Of course, she might feel that she is cheating if she only provides one session while she bills for two, but is there any moral reason why she should not provide the two?

Look at the case from the point of view of the third-party payor and those who have an interest in the funds in that insurance plan. A social utilitarian would want to get as much good as possible out of those funds. Presumably, the benefits should go to the subscribers who could get the most from the services. But should Ms. Dennelsten, a clinical care giver, be worried about the interests of the entire group of subscribers or only about the welfare of Mr. Lantress?

2. Benefits to Specific Nonpatients

A variant on the problem in the previous case arises when the allied health care worker can promote the interests of those other than the patient and those others are specific, identifiable nonpatients. These might be someone at risk from the patient of a threat of violence or an exposure to AIDS as in the following case.

CASE 14: Disclosing HIV Status: Do Nonpatients Have Claims?

Jack Jones is a 35-year-old executive with the California Technologies Corporation who has his eyes on the vice presidency

**This case was provided by Professor Ruth A. Hansen Ph.D., OTR.*

position that will become vacant in several months. He feels that his lover, Tom Lalli, chairman of the board, can be very influential in his getting the promotion. Very recently, Mr. Jones has been losing weight and tiring easily. He attributes these occurrences to the countless hours spent on the job in preparing for the anticipated promotion. Last week, he saw Todd Harrison, the physician assistant (PA), in the employee health unit for a bout of "short windedness." A series of tests were ordered, and today is a follow-up to that visit.

The PA greeted him politely and invited him into the office to share the test results. "Mr. Jones, as you may recall, one of the blood studies drawn last week was the ELISA test, which checks for the AIDS virus. Your results on this test were positive, which means you may have been exposed to the AIDS virus." After several minutes of silence and a panicky facial expression, Mr. Jones said, "Why I just can't believe it." The PA allowed him to express his feelings and recommended that he follow up with his private physician. The PA then said, "In the meantime, Mr. Jones, I suggest that every precaution be taken to prevent the spread of the virus and to inform your sexual partners of the test results." Mr. Jones' reply was, "Why, I can't do that, my career—my whole life is on the line." He then stormed out of the office.

As Mr. Jones left the office, the PA pondered what to do. He knew the patient's lover well; they had attended school together. After careful thought, the PA decided that it was his moral obligation to protect his friend, and he would therefore inform him of the test results.

Todd Harrison, the physician assistant in this case, faces a complex problem in calculating the possible benefits and harms of alternative courses of actions. What would be the potential harms and benefits to Jack Jones if Mr. Harrison discloses the HIV diagnosis to Tom Lalli, the corporation chairman? What would be the harms and benefits to the other parties?

The ethics of confidentiality will be explored in greater detail in the cases in Chapter 7. A preliminary problem needs to be addressed here. It seems likely that Mr. Jones has a great deal to lose and very little to gain by the disclosure. If the classical health care ethic that focuses exclusively on the welfare of the patient prevails, is there any reason for Mr. Harrison to disclose? On the other hand, newer versions of the ethics of the health professions consider the welfare of others at least under some circumstances. Is this one of those circumstances? If so, why? Does the fact that

Mr. Lalli can be identified make any moral difference? Compare this case to the two previous cases where it was clear that nonpatients had a lot to lose if allied health professionals did not speak out, but the allied health professional in those cases could not specifically identify who the victims would be. They were only statistics. Is the fact that Mr. Lalli can be identified morally significant? Is the fact that he is a long-term friend of Mr. Harrison's of any ethical significance?

3. Benefit to the Profession

One of the possible groups other than patients that could command the attention of the allied health professional is the professional group. It is the nature of a profession that its members perceive that they have an obligation to the professional group. It commands loyalty that requires certain sacrifices on the part of the individual. This is sometimes thought to include an obligation to conform to the moral standards of the profession, a problem addressed in the cases of the previous chapter. It also is sometimes believed to include a duty to promote the good of the profession. Since allied health professionals are traditionally thought to have a duty to promote the good of the patient, this raises an interesting problem when the good of the profession conflicts with the good of the patient. The following case poses the problem dramatically.

CASE 15: Striking to Benefit the Profession

Over the past year-and-a-half a group of health professionals at Adelphi University Hospital had been meeting with representatives of the administration in an attempt to resolve a series of complaints. The group consisted of members of the pharmacy, social work, respiratory care, physical therapy, laboratory, occupational therapy, and radiologic technology staffs. These individuals were members of an informal Professional Employees Association (PEA). Ginny Wadsworth, a respiratory care practitioner, had been active in this group.

The PEA was protesting a long-standing shortage of personnel in many departments resulting in forced overtime, high stress, and a poor working environment. They were also objecting to an administrative policy that placed a preference in hiring for nursing personnel. Further, there was a consensus that salary and benefits had not kept pace with those offered to professional employees at other institutions. Nonetheless, the group represented a loyal cadre of personnel who wished to resolve their complaints and remain at the institution.

During the course of the discussions, it became clear to the PEA that the issue of the working environment could be improved by more professional autonomy. The employees wanted greater responsibility and authority with respect to issues of professional practice, flexible scheduling, and personnel policies.

Unfortunately, the administration was unyielding in its position that the numbers of nursing personnel were of paramount importance and their belief that to delegate some of its authority for personnel policies was abrogation of its responsibility. This stance heightened tensions between the administration and PEA with the consequence that the PEA planned a series of job actions against the hospital.

Ginny Wadsworth was organizing the respiratory care practitioners to cooperate in a "prolonged education" session in which the PEA would confront the administration with their complaints. They agreed to be on call for emergencies, but refused to provide routine care. They knew the patients on the floor at the time would be at some risk, but they thought their profession and future patients would benefit in the long run. Did they do the right thing?

Here, Ginny Wadsworth and her colleagues are trading off the welfare of present patients for what they believe will be to long-term betterment of the profession and future patients. Exactly what do they mean when they say the job action will better the profession? Are they really saying that it will improve their pay? Or is the profession the beneficiary in some more subtle way? Is there a moral difference between taking a job action to better the profession and taking it to better the chances for future patients? Are the present patients more directly the moral responsibility of the health care workers contemplating the job action, or do future patients count just as much?

4. Benefit to the Allied Health Professional and His or Her Family

There is one final group of interests that could conflict with those of the patient: those of the allied health professional and his or her family. In the traditional Hippocratic health professional ethic, the only welfare that counted was that of the patient. There was never a formal recognition that the interests of the health professional could ever legitimately compete with those of the patient. Of course, health professionals have always recognized some limits to serving the patient. The following case explores those limits.

CASE 16: Risking HIV Exposure: May Self-interest Be Considered?

Rogers Memorial Hospital is a large urban institution located in a depressed neighborhood of poor, homeless, and IV drug users. For the protection of its employees as well as its patients, a policy of universal precautions was instituted. Blood and body fluid precautions are observed at all times for all patients.

At the time that the hospital established its AIDS unit, a policy was instituted that allowed professional staff to determine for themselves their willingness to be scheduled for work on the unit. For two years a sufficient number of volunteers was available to meet the personnel needs of the unit. However, staff turnover has resulted in a declining number of laboratory professionals willing to perform venipunctures on the unit.

Ms. Jennifer Williams, a medical technologist, has been volunteering to perform venipunctures on AIDS patients since the establishment of the unit. However, she has recently married and intends to become pregnant soon. Because she wants to do everything possible to ensure that she has a healthy baby, she no longer is willing to work on the AIDS unit.

Based upon epidemiologic data, which reveals no increased risk for health personnel working with AIDS patients, the hospital has modified its policy requiring rotational scheduling on the unit. Individuals no longer have the option of refusing to care for AIDS patients.

Because she worked voluntarily on the AIDS unit for two years, Ms. Williams believes that she should be exempt from the new policy. Further, she believes that her situation warrants an exemption. The health of her yet unborn child must take precedence over her obligation to provide her service to all patients.

Ms. Williams seems to have a case for being excused from further service on the AIDS unit. But ethically she still might ask what she ought to do. Suppose she considers only the welfare of her patients. Is she supposed to consider only her AIDS unit patients, or is it fair for her to consider the patients on the other units where she might work as well?

More critically, is it ethically legitimate for her to include in her calculation of the benefits and harms of alternative courses of action the effects on her and her unborn child? A utilitarian ethic will include consideration of all benefits and harms regardless of who is affected. That would include the benefits to herself and her child of avoiding the AIDS unit. Is it acceptable for a health professional to factor in her own welfare and that of family members when calculating benefits and harms?

Returning to consider the benefits and harms to the AIDS unit patients and the patients in the other units, if she decides to take the effects on both groups of patients into account, a utilitarian would insist that the only ethical course would be the one that maximized the net good considering both groups of patients. However, not everyone would agree that she should automatically choose the course that maximizes the total net good. She might, for example, give special weight to the fact that the AIDS patients (or some other patients) were particularly sick. Their need might give them a special claim to her attention even if following that course does not necessarily do the most good in aggregate. The cases in the following chapter force us to confront the question of whether special considerations such as need could be morally relevant in deciding how to allocate scarce health care resources such as time, energy, and money.

ENDNOTES

1. American Occupational Therapy Association (AOTA), *Occupational Therapy Code of Ethics*, 1994.
2. American Speech-Language-Hearing Association, *Code of Ethics*, published in *Asha*, Vol. 34 (March 1992), Suppl. 9, pp. 1-2.
3. American Academy of Physician Assistants (AAPA), House of Delegates, *Code of Ethics of the Physician Assistant Profession* (Alexandria, VA: AAPA, adopted 1983, amended 1985).
4. American Pharmaceutical Association, *Code of Ethics* (Washington, DC: APhA, 1981).
5. Jeremy Bentham, "An Introduction to the Principles of Morals and Legislation," in *Ethical Theories: A Book of Readings*, ed. I. Melden (Englewood Cliffs, NJ: Prentice Hall, 1967), pp. 367-390.
6. Milton C. Weinstein and William B. Stason, "Foundations of Cost-effectiveness Analysis for Health and Medical Practices," *The New England Journal of Medicine*, Vol. 296 (1977), pp. 716-721; R. M. Kaplan and J. W. Bush, "Health-Related Quality of Life Measurement for Evaluation Research and Policy Analysis," *Health Psychology*, Vol. 11 (1982), pp. 61-80; Abraham Mehrez and Amiram Gafni, "Quality-Adjusted Life Years, Utility Theory, and Healthy-Years Equivalents," *Medical Decision Making*, Vol. 9 (1989), pp. 142-149.

7. John Rawls, "Two Concepts of Rules," *The Philosophical Review*, Vol. 44 (1955), pp. 3-32, and David Lyons, *Forms and Limits of Utilitarianism* (Oxford: Oxford University Press, 1965).
8. AOTA, *Occupational Therapy Code of Ethics*.
9. AAPA, *Code of Ethics of the Physician Assistant Profession*. (Alexandria, VA)

CHAPTER 4

Justice

THE ALLOCATION OF HEALTH RESOURCES

In the previous chapter when the principles of beneficence and nonmaleficence—of doing good and avoiding harm—were introduced one of the problems raised was the conflict between the welfare of the patient and the welfare of other parties. The utilitarian solution to this problem is to strive to maximize the total amount of good that was done regardless of who the beneficiary is. We saw that sometimes that conflicted with the Hippocratic ethic, which requires that the health professional focus exclusively on the welfare of the patient.

Allied health professionals often find themselves in situations in which the interests of their patients are in conflict. They must choose between clients or between a client and those who are not clients. Whether to spend a long time with one terribly sick patient or shorter, more efficient sessions with several relatively healthier ones is one example. Whether to provide care for a patient who obviously cannot pay knowing that others will, in effect, cover the costs is another. The Hippocratic mandate to serve the interests of the patient (in the singular) does not help. On the other hand, it seems ethically crass simply to count up the total amounts of good and harm and choose the course that maximizes total social outcome regardless of the impact on the individuals affected. That could lead, for instance, to refusing to provide services to those who are not useful to society or to those who cannot themselves benefit greatly from the health care provider's services.

Some ethical theories introduce a new ethical principle to deal with this problem—the principle of justice.[1] While beneficence and nonmaleficence are devoted, respectively, simply to producing as much good and preventing as much harm as possible, justice is concerned with how the goods and harms are distributed. Justice is concerned with the equity or fairness of the patterns of the benefits and harms.

Among those who hold that there is a principle of justice that is concerned about the ways goods and harms are distributed, there are many schools of thought regarding what counts as a just or equitable distribution.

The just distribution might focus on the effort of the various parties (even if sometimes those exerting great effort do not produce beneficial outcomes). Others emphasize entitlements based on ownership, so that one is entitled to whatever one has acquired provided it has been obtained without coercion.[2] Still others, especially in health care, look at the need of the parties.[3]

In health care, those who are in the greatest need (those who are the sickest) may not be the most efficient to treat. In such cases, a choice must be made between using health care services in the way that will do the most good (sometimes treating healthier, more stable patients) and treating those with the greatest need. Any ethical principle that focuses on maximizing the good done for patients would tolerate—indeed require—that those with the greatest need be sacrificed. On the other hand, a principle of justice that focuses on need would accept the inefficiencies of an allocation of health resources that concentrates on the neediest. The cases in this chapter look at various problems of health resource allocation and the conflict between maximizing efficiency called for by the principles of beneficence and nonmaleficence and distributing resources equitably called for by the principle of justice.

JUSTICE AMONG CLIENTS

Some allied health professionals accept the traditional Hippocratic ethic that limits the focus of ethical responsibility to the welfare of the patient. They hold that it is simply outside the moral scope of the provider's role to worry about saving society money, catching welfare cheaters, or serving other societal interests.

Even the Hippocratic health care provider sometimes still must allocate resources. He or she may face a direct conflict between the interests of different patients. The next two cases raise such conflicts.

CASE 17: Need Versus Benefit: Choosing Between Patients

Sue Herriot is the manager of the Occupational Therapy Department in an acute care setting. Today is Friday. Five new referrals are received for occupational therapy. But, because of short staffing, only one patient can be seen. Prioritization of the patients' needs allows her to defer three, but two patients should be seen today. Who should be chosen? Keep in mind that the weekend is coming up and occupational therapy services are not available.

Donald Wachsman was admitted five days ago following a right-hemisphere cerebrovascular accident (CVA). Mrs. Herriot learns from the physical therapist (PT) that the patient has excellent rehabilitation potential because his left arm and leg are not completely flaccid. Furthermore, Mr. Wachsman has a supportive family. The physicians have been trying, so far unsuccessfully, to get the patient admitted to a rehabilitation unit before the last four Diagnosis Related Group (DRG) days run out. Mrs. Herriot realizes that Mr. Wachsman will probably do fairly well even without her services, but she is sure she could do him a great deal of good.

Gertrude Finnerty is an elderly woman admitted five days ago with a hip fracture. The social work report notes that this woman lives alone in the country and has no close relatives. A psychiatric consultation report indicates that Mrs. Finnerty has dementia. It questions the patient's ability to return to her home and live alone, but says that the patient herself is determined to do so. There are six DRG days left. Mrs. Herriot feels how desperate this woman is and wants to respond to her need, but realizes she probably is not going to help her as much as she could help Mr. Wachsman. Whom should she treat?

In the previous chapter, cases were analyzed to determine the total net benefits (the benefits minus the harms) of alternative courses of actions. We distinguished between medical and nonmedical benefits. We also distinguished between calculating benefits based on individual cases and based on the general rule. Based on the determination of benefits and harms, would more good be done treating Mr. Wachsman or Mrs. Finnerty? Does this assessment hold up considering both psychological and medical benefits that Mrs. Herriot could offer the two patients?

Mrs. Herriot seems to believe that she can do more good for Mr. Wachsman. Does that settle the matter morally? According to a utilitarian it would, but why is Mrs. Herriot considering treating Mrs. Finnerty? It appears that she is worse off; her need is greater than Mr. Wachsman's even though Mrs. Herriot probably can do her less good.

One version of the principle of justice holds that an action is morally right insofar as it benefits those whose need is greatest. According to one version of this position, the goal is to improve the lot of the worst off. This is called the "maximin" view; the goal is to maximize the minimum *even if doing so does not maximize the total amount of good done*.[4] A slightly different interpretation of the principle of justice holds that an action is right insofar as it makes the distribution of benefits more equal.[5] Who would get Mrs. Herriot's attention under these interpretations of the principle of justice?

Assuming that Mrs. Herriot can do more good by helping Mr. Wachsman, but that Mrs. Finnerty is in greater need, how should Mrs. Herriot balance these competing claims on her time?

CASE 18: Criteria for Allocation: Time, Age, Need, and Benefit

Jill Johnson is the only physical therapist working during the lunch hour in the Rehab Clinic. At 12 noon, Richard Sims, a 37-year-old male who has recently had arthroplastic surgery on his left knee, arrives right on time for knee-strengthening exercises therapy. Mr. Sims injured his knee playing racquet ball.

At 12:05 P.M. Arlene Goldson is brought into the clinic on a plinth. Mrs. Goldson, who is 89 years old, recently suffered a CVA. She also is diabetic and has congestive heart failure. Mrs. Goldson was supposed to have arrived at 11:00 A.M. in physical therapy, but due to a mixup with the escort service, she doesn't appear until 12:05 P.M.

To make matters worse, Christopher Farrar, a 16-year-old male, comes into the clinic at 12:07. He is scheduled for noon to receive gait training. Christopher has just had "in and out" surgery to remove a bunion from his right foot. Christopher is anxious to leave. His mother is waiting to take him home. They live 50 miles away.

Much to Jill Johnson's dismay, all the other therapists have gone out for lunch. Jill's dilemma is who should be treated first. Normal protocol provides that patients who are the sickest or in the most distress are supposed to be seen first. At the same time, patients who arrive on time are supposed to have priority.

Just as Ms. Johnson figures out in her mind how she is going to handle this situation, Mr. Frank Holman, a 71-year-old seriously debilitated emphysema patient, comes into the clinic in a wheel chair. He is supposed to receive chest physical therapy. His appointment isn't until 1:00 P.M., but he is acutely uncomfortable. Ms. Johnson hates to make him wait.

Whom should Ms. Johnson treat first and why?

Look at the case first from the straightforward utilitarian perspective. Which patient would be benefited most by being given first priority? Does the relief given to an impatient Christopher and his mother count as a legitimate benefit? If Mrs. Goldson were the least rushed and had the most time to spare, should Ms. Johnson place her at the end of the list on the grounds that she will be hurt the least by waiting? Should Mr. Holman go to the front of the line because he will suffer the most if he waits?

How would the principle of justice modify Ms. Johnson's decision? The versions of justice examined in the previous case give priority to the one who is worst off. Who would get priority on this basis?

These patients are very different in their ages. What role, if any, should age play in deciding priorities? What role should the appointments of the patients play? Should Mrs. Goldson's late arrival be a factor that would count against her? Should Mr. Holman's early arrival be a reason to have him wait until his appointment time? Should Christopher Farrar and Richard Sims get first priority based on appointment time? Is an allied health professional responsible for managing time or patient cases? In an era where reimbursement is so critical, how do factors of patient case management and reimbursement interface?

JUSTICE BETWEEN CLIENTS AND OTHERS

In both of the previous cases, clients were competing among themselves for scarce resources—an allied health professional's time that can only go to one patient in the first case, a place in line in the second. Sometimes, however, a client is competing with others who are not clients. An allied health professional must choose between the client and others. Of course, we saw in Chapter 3 that in purely Hippocratic ethics, the client is the only interest that is morally relevant. According to the Hippocratic ethic, the health care provider has a duty to totally ignore the interests of others. The following cases make clear that sometimes that is hard to do.

CASE 19: Justice Between Clients and Others

Janet Howard is a physical therapist who is employed by the Capitol Home Health Care Agency. The agency has a contract with the Golden Age Senior Citizen Center. Ms. Howard has a standing appointment with Mrs. Vera Green to provide gait training. Mrs. Green had a mild stroke 11 months ago. Since then she has had physical therapy to improve her ability to walk about and to increase her endurance.

On Thursdays, Ms. Howard treats Mrs. Green from 3:00 to 4:00 P.M. and then has to pick up her son at a day care center by 4:30 P.M. On a particular Thursday, Ms. Howard arrives at the senior citizen center to provide gait training. On her way into the center, Ms. Howard encounters another senior citizen, Mrs. Marian Branch, who has fallen in the lobby. She is not a patient of Ms. Howard's, but she has seen her at the center before. It is commonly known that Mrs. Branch has been suffering from vertigo.

Given the fact that Ms. Howard is running about 15 minutes late, stopping to administer assistance to Mrs. Branch would completely throw her schedule off. To complicate matters, Janet Howard has had a very sore back for the past several days. Helping Mrs. Branch up would be harmful to her back condition.

Questions for Discussion

1. Using the criterion of opting for the course that will do the most good, what would Ms. Howard choose?
2. Using the principle of justice (interpreted as priority for the worst off), what would she choose?
3. If Mrs. Branch wins on both criteria, what should Mrs. Howard make of the fact that only Mrs. Green is her patient and that she is late to see her?
4. If Ms. Howard could help both a patient and a nonpatient equally, is there any reason to give priority to the patient?
5. What role should the interests of Ms. Howard's son play in her decision?
6. Under what conditions, if any, should she delay helping a patient to help a nonpatient? Would the fact that she could benefit Mrs. Branch more justify the delay? Would the fact that Mrs. Branch is worse off than Mrs. Green?

Similar questions apply to the following cases:

CASE 20: Prolonged Treatment of a Hopeless Case: Is It Fair?

At the time of his accident, Jay Marrow was 36 years old, an employed stepfather of four teenagers. He sustained a severe brain injury in a motor vehicle accident (MVA) in which one of his teenage stepsons was killed.

Mr. Marrow has had a long and stormy rehabilitation course. He received physical and occupational therapy. His improvement, both physically and cognitively, was slow and very limited. He had gait impairment and severe fine motor problems. The motor problems have limited Mr. Marrow's ability to perform basic self-care activities independently. Cognitively, he has shown total loss of all abstracting skills: his judgment impaired, ability to reason gone, planning and sequencing skills at approximately chronological age 2 years. He has lost the ability to interpret time sequences and he experiences memories of remote events with the same emotional impact as immediate ones. He could not process any new information for many months. He finally grasped the fact of the death of his stepson and was grief stricken and angry at his wife for not "giving a damn." It took many weeks for the staff and family to convince him that his wife had grieved too for her son.

Mr. Marrow was discharged to his home. In a very short period of time it became clear that he could not be managed at home. The extent of the cognitive, ambulation, and self-care problems, similar to that of a 2-year-old but on a 6′5″, 240-pound frame, made home management dangerous. In desperation the wife requested readmittance to the state-run rehabilitation center, and he was accepted.

Over the next several months every effort was made to find appropriate placement for Mr. Marrow in a facility that his insurance would cover. After literally dozens of letters, justifications, and denials, this effort dead-ended. Physically and emotionally, Mr. Marrow had progressed to the point that hospital rehab was completely unsatisfactory. He grew more angry and depressed daily. Cognitively, he desperately needed to continue his OT program. There was no insurance coverage for outpatient services; his income was sufficient only for sheltered living costs. If discharged from the hospital, his OT ended; yet he was totally unwilling to stay in the hospital to get therapy. Worse, his insurance company, after 18 months, had notified the rehab center that his coverage would be terminated in the near future.

Mr. Marrow has created an ethical problem for the rehab center because he is clearly in need of extensive care. Moreover, all sources of funding of that care seem to be gone. It appears that no one is going to reimburse the rehab center; it will have to absorb the considerable costs. But in doing so either resources (time, energy, and money) will have to be diverted from other patients, or additional funds will have to be provided. Even if the rehab center could persuade the state to increase its appropriation, that would simply divert the problem since the state would have to transfer funds from some other worthwhile project.

Given the intense effort required to show even modest progress with Mr. Marrow, it seems clear that more good could be done with the resources used in other ways either within the rehab center or in other state projects. Nevertheless, Mr. Marrow is surely among the neediest, worst-off citizens of the state. Should the state maximize its efficiency getting the most net good per unit of investment (even if it means warehousing some unfortunate severely handicapped citizens), or should it purposely decide (appealing to the principle of justice rather than utility) to decrease the total good it can do so as to give special attention to its least-well-off citizens?

CASE 21: Scarce Resources

A local rehabilitation center with strict criteria for admissions had all its beds filled. Each department had to demonstrate the efficacy of its treatment and had to produce enough income to warrant increased staffing.

The Occupational Therapy Department is composed of the director, one senior therapist, three staff therapists, and one certified occupational therapy assistant (COTA). The average patient load per therapist was 12 daily. The primary focus of treatment was self care, communication, mobility, work hardening, community living skills, and driver training. Shirley Harrison, director of the Department of Occupational Therapy, received a telephone call from one of her staff therapists who had recently been in an automobile accident. The therapist's doctor had prescribed light duty only with no lifting, pushing, or pulling for the next six weeks. The hospital's policy was that employees injured other than on the job could not come back to work until they received a medical release for full duty. Mrs. Harrison supervises another therapist in her fifth month of a very difficult pregnancy. The workload in occupational therapy has already been adjusted to allow the pregnant therapist to assume some administrative and quality assurance duties.

This decrease of human resources had caused an extensive waiting list for occupational therapy. Mrs. Harrison felt very bad about denying or postponing treatment to previously screened patients deserving services. Many of these patients had come from great distances and had family support and other nonmedical factors that might affect their rehabilitative potential.

Mrs. Harrison's immediate supervisor had stated that she could not have the staff therapist who was in the automobile accident return because it was against hospital policy. Yet the department was losing income, and the patients' rehabilitation was being compromised. She was being pushed to maintain her department's productivity level and had assumed a patient case load as a way of trying to maintain the numbers. Mrs. Harrison also felt that to push her overworked staff to do more would jeopardize the quality of patient care.*

Questions for Discussion

1. Is it equitable to place one therapist informally on light duty and have another not be able to return to work because of hospital policy?
2. How should the shortcomings of services be addressed?
3. How should the larger problem of staffing tied to generated income be addressed?
4. How do the selection criteria used to admit patients to this rehabilitation services facility affect decision making?
5. How should the facility's obligation to provide comprehensive rehabilitation services affect decision making concerning staff shortages?
6. Does the patient's right to the expectation of comprehensive rehabilitation services affect provision of services?
7. What future harm, if any, can be done by providing minimal occupational therapy services to patients expecting occupational therapy?

JUSTICE AND LIFE-STYLE HEALTH RISKS

Increasingly the ethics of the distribution of scarce resources must deal with the fact that some patients need health care because of their voluntary choices in their life-styles. Alcoholics, overweight heart attack victims, smokers, and substance abusers all can create medical problems for themselves by their behavior. It is often difficult to determine whether their behavior is really voluntary, but to the extent that it is, questions are raised

**This case was contributed by Professor Ruth Hansen Ph.D., OTR.*

about whether it is equitable or just to devote community health care resources toward their self-inflicted medical needs.

Many people hold that health professionals should ignore this in deciding who is entitled to health care either because it is so difficult to determine whether the behavior is truly voluntary or simply because health professionals have a duty to respond to need when it is encountered.[6] Others, however, are beginning to consider life-style choices morally relevant in allocating scarce resources.[7] Does the voluntary behavior of the client in the following case affect his moral right of access to a health care provider's services?

CASE 22: Therapy or Prison: Do Life-style Choices Negate a Right to Therapy?

Kenny Smith is a single, 19-year-old, Baptist male who was born and raised in Detroit. He was convicted in Detroit City Circuit Court of grand larceny-auto and possession of burglary tools. He was given a six-year suspended prison term in the state penitentiary and was mandated to participate in a rehabilitation program for one year. He is required to remain in the agency's residential program for 60 days; then he must return to live with his parents while he continues his participation in the program. Mr. Smith is very close to his parents and sister, as they are his major support system. Mr. Smith has a residential case manager to whom he reports daily, and Janice Rothman, the program social worker, sees him on a weekly basis for intensive supervision. This supervision includes the monitoring of Mr. Smith's treatment-behavioral plan, which is mandated by the court/judge, and in-depth counseling. The main goal at this time is for Mr. Smith to successfully complete his treatment plan.

Ethical Issue: The problem in this case concerns the discrepancy between the client's treatment needs and the agency's rules and regulations. Mr. Smith had initially stated in the intake reports that he had experimented with marijuana in the past and used alcohol occasionally. According to his treatment plan, he is required to submit to random urine screens in the residential facility. It is the rule of the facility that if a client receives two positive urines, he or she is returned to prison.

Mr. Smith has just received his second positive urine for alcohol, and the staff is considering sending him back to prison. As a professional social worker, Ms. Rothman believes that if Mr. Smith returns to prison, his drug problem will not be addressed. She feels it would be more beneficial for him to continue in the program so they could address and work on the problem through individual treatment. In addition, Mr. Smith has disclosed in a confidential counseling session that he recently bought another client's urine (someone he knew was drug free) to avoid another violation.

Question for Discussion

1. Should Ms. Rothman support the staff's decision to send Mr. Smith back to prison when she knows that his continuance in the program is more beneficial for his treatment needs?

It seems clear that Mr. Smith could benefit from the social worker's continuing interventions. On the grounds of patient benefit, Ms. Rothman's duty would be to do what she can to make sure he continues in therapy. Likewise, the principle of justice, insofar as it requires giving priority to those who have the greatest need, probably would support continued therapy for him. But justice is a complex principle. In general, it looks at the pattern of the distribution of benefits and harms. While need is one criterion of just allocation, it is not the only one. Some people consider distributions of resources solely based on effort or merit, others according to chance. The issue raised in this case is whether Mr. Smith's behavior was voluntary and whether it should influence Mr. Smith's right to therapy from health care providers.

JUSTICE IN PUBLIC POLICY

The questions of justice in the allocation of resources arise not only in clinical situations, but also in matters of policy. A key difference is that the allied health professional facing policy decisions does not have a specific patient or patients in mind whose interests can be served. If a specific patient's case is debated, it is as an example of a more general policy question in which the interests of a group are at stake, as the health maintenance organization (HMO) subscribers in the following case, or in a community whose interests must be treated fairly. The health professional in such cases is not so much acting as an agent for the specific patient as for the entire group.

CASE 23: Equity or Efficiency in Community Public Health Programs

Donna Hatwick is a dental hygienist who is a specialist in the use of dental sealants (polymer compounds placed on children's teeth to prevent dental caries). She works in school health programs for the White County Health Department. She knows that research indicates that the use of sealants for 12-year-old school children dramatically reduces cavities.[8]

The county health department has a modest budget ($20,000) for all the children in the county, not nearly enough to seal all children's teeth. The public health dentistry division of the department has to make a policy decision. Which children should get the sealants? Should they go to the children in the schools in the lowest-income areas? Should they be distributed by lot?

A technical complication suggests another possibility. Dental sealants prevent caries primarily on the occlusal (flat biting) surfaces of the teeth. However, if there are cavities on the interstitial surfaces between the teeth, the dentist must destroy the seal to do a restoration of the cavity.

Donna Hatwick and her colleagues in the dentistry division know that fluoride prevents primarily interstitial cavities. Thus, sealants are much more efficient when combined with fluoride treatment.

They also realize that certain communities in the county have fluoridated water while others do not. Therefore, if they want to get the maximum reduction of dental caries for their $20,000 invested in sealants, they could use the funds to provide sealants with priority for those communities that have fluoridated water.

Ms. Hatwick's problem is that even though she knows that giving priority to children in communities with fluoridated water is efficient, she is not sure that such a decision would be fair. Whatever anyone thinks about fluoridated water, it is surely not the children's fault if they live in communities that do not fluoridate. Is it ethical to deprive those children of the benefits of sealants? Moreover, she knows that some of those children in communities without fluoride have parents who have taken steps to make sure their children get fluoride (through use of fluoride toothpaste or with fluoride treatments from private dentists). Thus, they would actually get the full benefit of the sealants. Still, Ms. Hatwick realizes they are running a community school-based program. There is no way they can provide sealants to individual children whose teeth have received fluoride. If they want to get maximum benefit from their investment they will arbitrarily use their funds in the communities with the fluoride. Should they strive for maximum efficiency or should they lower the efficiency to give all children an equal chance to get the fluoride treatment?

This is a classic case of having to choose between the principle of beneficence (maximizing the net good in aggregate) and the principle of justice (interpreted as treating people equally). Assuming that it is not possible to get enough funds appropriated to provide sealants for all the 12-year-old children in the county, the department must choose who gets the priority and what ethical principle should govern.

JUSTICE AND OTHER ETHICAL PRINCIPLES

We have, throughout this chapter, been examining how the principle of justice relates to the principles of beneficence and nonmaleficence. Nonutilitarians hold that there are right-making characteristics of actions other than the net amount of good produced that are morally relevant. Justice, which is some morally right pattern of the distribution of benefits and burdens, is just one such principle of rightness. In later chapters other principles that are sometimes identified as right-making characteristics will be discussed. These include respect for autonomy, truth-telling, fidelity to promises, and the duty to avoid killing. We shall see that sometimes these come into conflict. When they do, a full ethic will have to have some method for resolving the conflict. One approach is to view each principle (right-making characteristic) as an element that will tend to make actions right. Then considering only the single dimension, the action is right. It would be right if there were no conflicting considerations pulling in the other direction. When ethical principles are used to identify these right-making elements, they are called *prima facie* principles. They identify characteristics that would make an action right "other things being equal." In the following case, we can identify what justice requires, but we might also have to take into account that certain commitments have been made that would pull the therapist in the other direction. Here is an example of a conflict between the principles of justice and fidelity.

CASE 24: Quality Versus Quantity

Mary Koopman has been working as an occupational therapist in a mental health facility for five years. In that time she has worked almost exclusively with patients in group sessions. She has been seeing three groups of 10-12 patients each day, some of whom she has been working with for as long as two years. She has found that this is the maximum number of patients and number of groups that she can handle and provide quality treatment.

Recently there has been a great increase in the number of patients being admitted to her facility. As a result she has many more referrals for group therapy. Some of the new patients seem much worse off than the patients she has been seeing regularly. She could see as many as 60 patients a day if she had the time. Ms. Koopman has asked administration for more staff to assist with therapy, but because of budget constraints she has been told that no one can be hired. She wonders whether she should cut back on her more established patients to help those in greater need or whether, when she established a professional relation with the first patients, she made a commitment to them that she shouldn't break.

Probably Ms. Koopman would take the new patients if she were guided solely by the principle of beneficence. Is it clear that she would do more good by doing so? Likewise, if the principle of justice were her guiding principle and justice were interpreted as directing benefit to the worse off, she would probably shift her attention to the new patients, at least the ones who were in greater need.

If this seems right, then why does she feel any reluctance to shift? Maximizing the good (beneficence) is one characteristic of actions that makes them right. If there were no other considerations, certainly it would be morally better to choose the course that will do the most good. Likewise, distributing benefits to help those in greatest need is a characteristic of actions that many people believe makes them right.

These are not the only right-making characteristics, however. Another principle that identifies a characteristic that tends to make actions right is fidelity to promises. If Ms. Koopman has an obligation to her earlier patients, it must be a duty of fidelity—based on an implied promise she made that she will remain with them (even if there are moral reasons to go on to others).

Thus, even if it is clear what beneficence or justice requires, the ethical work in resolving the case problem is not finished. A full ethical theory will also have to have an answer to the question of what should be done when various ethical principles come into conflict.

One possibility is to try to rank the principles. Can beneficence, justice, or fidelity to promises categorically be ranked highest? If not, another possibility is that once the various principles are identified, they are "balanced" making a case-by-case judgment as to which principle wins out.

Still a third possibility is that maximizing net benefits must morally give way to the result of "balancing" of the other principles. In that case, whenever there was only one other principle at stake or when consideration of all other principles gave a clear answer, beneficence would not come into play. However, in cases where two other principles neutralized each other or when no other principles were at stake, then beneficence and nonmaleficence would come into play. The cases in the next four chapters introduce, respectively, the principles of autonomy, veracity, fidelity, and avoidance of killing.

ENDNOTES

1. For some of the important literature on justice and health resource allocation, see President's Commission for the Study of Ethical Problems in Medicine and Biomedical and Behavioral Research, *Securing Access to Health Care,* Vol. 1 (Washington, DC: U.S. Government Printing Office, 1983); Paul Menzel, *Strong Medicine: The Ethical Rationing of Health Care* (New York: Oxford University Press, 1990); Norman Daniels, *Just Health Care* (Cambridge: Cambridge University Press, 1985); and Daniel Callahan, *What Kind of Life: The Limits of Medical Progress* (New York: Simon & Schuster, 1990).
2. H. Tristram Engelhardt, *The Foundations of Bioethics* (New York: Oxford University Press, 1986).
3. Ronald M. Green, "Health Care and Justice in Contract Theory Perspective," in *Ethics and Health Policy,* ed. Robert M. Veatch and Roy Branson (Cambridge, MA: Ballinger, 1976); Robert M. Veatch, *The Foundations of Justice: Why the Retarded and the Rest of Us Have Claims to Equality* (New York: Oxford University Press, 1986).
4. John Rawls, *A Theory of Justice* (Cambridge, MA: Harvard University Press, 1971).

5. Veatch, *The Foundations of Justice.*
6. Dan E. Beauchamp, "Public Health as Social Justice," *Inquiry,* Vol. 13 (1976), pp. 3-14.
7. Robert M. Veatch, "Voluntary Risks to Health: The Ethical Issues," *Journal of the American Medical Association,* Vol. 243 (January 4, 1980), pp. 50-55.
8. National Institutes of Health, "Consensus Development Conference Statement: Dental Sealants in the Prevention of Tooth Decay," *Journal of Dental Education,* Vol. 48 (February 1984), Suppl., pp. 126-131.

CHAPTER 5

Autonomy

In the previous chapter we saw that in social ethics the principles of beneficence and nonmaleficence (maximizing aggregate total net benefits) may not be the only morally relevant consideration. The principle of justice affirms that certain patterns of distribution of the good, such as distribution based on medical need, may also be morally relevant. Justice in distribution is not the only moral consideration that can provide a check on the principles of beneficence and nonmaleficence. In this and the following chapters, we shall explore several other moral principles—autonomy, veracity, fidelity, and avoidance of killing—principles that all, in one way or another, refer to right-making elements of actions or practices that do not focus on maximizing the net good produced.

Justice is concerned with the distribution of goods in morally preferred patterns. It, therefore, always involves more than one person who is the potential beneficiary. The remaining principles are relevant, however, even if there is only one person our actions affect. Thus, these principles are particularly important in traditional clinical health care ethics in which the professional is thought of as acting on one and only one patient. In fact, we increasingly recognize that even in these clinical situations many people are affected by the clinician's actions. There is not only one patient, but other patients whom the clinician could be treating. There are family members of the patient, friends, and citizens affected by each treatment decision as well as fellow health professionals whose lives are affected.

Nevertheless, many ethical decisions in health care can be analyzed as if there were only one party who was principally affected. When we contemplate violating a patient's autonomy, lying to a patient, breaking a promise such as the promise of confidentiality, or acting in a way that will kill a patient, it is the patient's moral interests that are primarily affected. Other people's interests are much more indirect. Therefore, while remembering the important ethical issues raised by the principle of justice in the previous chapter, the cases in this and the following chapters in this parc of the book will focus primarily on the more individual ethical concerns. These begin with the moral principle of autonomy.[1]

Autonomy is both a psychological and a moral term. Psychologically, autonomy is a term describing the mental state of persons who are free to choose their own life plans and act on those plans substantially independent of internal or external constraints. One leads the life of an autonomous person to the extent that one is free to be "self-legislating." Autonomy means creating one's own legislation. As such, it should be apparent that being autonomous is always a matter of degree. No one is "fully autonomous" in the sense of being totally free from internal and external constraints. Some people may be totally lacking in autonomy—infants and the comatose are examples. However, many people who we think of as lacking autonomy possess some limited capacity to make their own choices. Small children, the mentally retarded, the mentally ill, and the senile all may be able to make limited choices based on their own beliefs and values and yet are hardly autonomous enough to be called self-determining in any meaningful way. Thus being an autonomous person is a matter of degree. Those persons who have a sufficient degree of autonomy we treat as being essentially self-determining; we could call them "substantially autonomous persons."

For purposes of public policy, we assume that persons below the age of majority, usually 18, are lacking sufficient autonomy for a range of publicly significant decisions unless proven otherwise. We admit that some 16-year-olds may have both the internal knowledge and intellectual capacity and be sufficiently free from external constraints to be as autonomous as some adults. The courts will occasionally recognize such minors as "mature" for purposes of making medical decisions on their own. But the working presumption is that minors lack competence to make many substantially autonomous decisions.

On the other hand, those who have reached the age of majority are presumed to be substantially autonomous unless there is adequate evidence to the contrary. One kind of evidence comes from a judicial determination of lack of competence. There is a striking problem with many patients who are clearly unconscious or semiconscious. They are obviously not capable of making autonomous decisions, yet they have never been declared incompetent. One approach is to require anyone who believes such persons are totally lacking in competence to make the needed decisions to take reasonable steps to inform the patient of this belief. If the patient disagrees, then he or she should be presumed to be competent until a court determines otherwise. If he or she fails to disagree, then it seems reasonable to presume that patient lacks the capacity to make substantially autonomous choices. Some patients will not disagree because they concur in the judgment that they are not competent; others because they are incapable of responding coherently.[2]

This, however, does not mean automatically that a clinical care giver is free to do what seems reasonable to those who are not substantially autonomous. In the case of children, we presume only parents and those designated by the courts may legitimately act as surrogate decision makers. In the case of adults, even if the presumption of lack of autonomy is warranted, we still need to determine who is authorized to speak for the individual. The health professional—allied health professional, physician, or other health worker—does not automatically have that authority.

On the other hand, even if one is believed to be substantially autonomous, it does not necessarily follow that he or she should be free to make all decisions about his or her actions. If one's actions are likely to harm others, we often accept the idea that they can be restrained. This might be supported on what can be called the "harm to others" principle. This is simply the principle that someone's autonomy can be constrained when that person's behavior risks causing harm to others. From the time of John Stuart Mill, this limit on action has been well recognized, even among defenders of human liberty.[3] The principle of justice might also be a basis for constraining actions that affect others. That is, we may want to control people because of the effect of their actions on the distribution of goods as well as because of the total amount of benefits and harms their actions will bring to others.

Even if one's substantially autonomous actions have no appreciable effect on other people, it is still an open question whether it is ethically right to permit people to make choices about their own lives. Even if an individual's free choices affect only that individual, some people have held that it is morally appropriate to constrain actions in order to protect the individual from himself. This is where autonomy surfaces as a *moral* principle. The moral principle of autonomy holds that an action or practice is morally wrong insofar as it attempts to control the actions of substantially autonomous persons on the basis of a concern for their own welfare.

Classical Hippocratic ethics in the health care professions has been committed to the principle that the health care worker should do whatever is necessary to benefit the patient. This has been understood to include violating the autonomy of the patient. Health care workers in the name of Hippocratic paternalism have refused to tell patients the names of drugs they were taking, restrained patients using Posey belts and bed rails, forced them to eat, used placebo treatments, and engaged in all manner of violations of the autonomous choices of patients. They have done so not out of a concern to protect the welfare of others or to promote justice, but rather out of concern that the patient would hurt himself or herself. Classical Hippocratic professional ethics contains no moral principle of autonomy.

By contrast, the moral principle of autonomy says that patients have a right to be self-determining insofar as their actions affect only themselves. The principle of autonomy poses increasingly difficult moral problems for allied health professionals, first, in determining whether patients really are sufficiently autonomous that the principle of respect for autonomy applies; second, in deciding whether persons who are, in principle, sufficiently autonomous are being constrained by external forces that control their choices; and, third, in deciding whether it is morally appropriate to override autonomy in order to protect the welfare of the patient. For example, the *Occupational Therapy Code of Ethics* (revised in 1994) says that OTs "shall respect the individual's right to refuse professional services," but also "shall take all reasonable precautions to avoid harm to the recipient of services."[4] Both of these appear in a section labeled "Beneficence/autonomy." However, the first provision seems to be supported by the principle of autonomy (even though it might violate the principle of beneficence), while the second seems to be supported by the principle of beneficence (even though it might violate the principle of autonomy). The following cases confront these issues.

DETERMINING WHETHER A PATIENT IS AUTONOMOUS

First, some persons may lack the capacity to make many substantially autonomous decisions. They may, through age or brain pathology, lack the neurological capacity to process information necessary for making choices. They may suffer from severe mental impairments, delusions, or errors in understanding.

In the easy cases, this capacity is totally lacking. It is these cases, such as with small children, in which we presume by public policy that autonomy is absent and designate someone as a surrogate, such as a parent or court-appointed guardian. For adults in whom autonomy appears to be totally lacking, matters are more complex. First, the adult may have made choices while competent that are thought to be still relevant. Second, decisions may have been made by a third party while an individual was incompetent. Third, there is no way to automatically assume incompetence (as with someone under the age of majority). It is here that we are still striving to develop legal and public policy mechanisms for transferring decision-making authority.[5]

There is presently no clear legal authority for health professionals, on their own, to declare incompetency and assume the role of surrogate decision maker. Competence is a legal term that can be determined only by the courts. Since adults are normally presumed competent until adjudicated otherwise, there is a real problem for adults in need of medical treatment who appear to lack capacity for making autonomous choices and yet need medical treatment immediately. There is a legal "presumption of consent" in cases of emergency.[6] That presumption is not valid, however, for situations that are not emergencies such as planning to write a medical order not to resuscitate a patient in the case of a cardiac arrest. It is also probably not valid for emergencies in which the patient is coherent enough to demand not to be treated. As a society we are moving toward a consensus that in cases in which the patient is so lacking in capacity he or she cannot respond coherently to a declaration of incompetency, the transfer of decision making to the appropriate surrogate is acceptable, even without a formal court review. Still that leaves open the question of who the appropriate surrogate should be. The pattern emerging seems to be that it is the next of kin rather than the health professional in charge as it was formerly assumed in many instances.

In cases in which the patient can respond to a declaration of lack of capacity by the care provider, it is much less clear what should be done. If there is enough time, it is probably best to seek informal help from an ethics committee or formal, legally binding review from a court. If there is not enough time, it is far less clear what should be done.

1. Autonomy in Adolescents

One group of patients who pose the problem of whether they are sufficiently autonomous to make their own medical decisions is the adolescent, particularly the adolescent who suffers some degree of mental impairment.

CASE 25: May a Mature Minor Refuse Life-Sustaining Treatment?

Jimmy Scott is a 12-year-old young man who is remarkably mature for his years. He is suffering from cystic fibrosis and is currently being treated in Children's Hospital. His life expectancy is probably less than one year. He understands that his condition is very serious and that he is not expected to live beyond the next several months.

His physical therapist is Ted Young, who generally has great rapport with difficult patients. For the past week, when Mr. Young has attempted to treat Jimmy with postural drainage therapy, he has gone into tantrums and refused the treatment.

Jimmy's parents are ambivalent about the situation. They would desperately like to see Jimmy live, but understand the limited possibilities and hate to see him suffer endlessly. They reluctantly are willing to support their son's decision.

Should Mr. Young take steps to override Jimmy's refusal? In this case, Jimmy's prognosis is not good. Even though he is clearly a minor, the complicating factor of his mental maturity raises an interesting dilemma for the allied health professional. Is it in Jimmy's best interest to seek to override his refusal of treatment and, if so, should Mr. Young attempt to do so? Or is the terminal nature of his condition coupled with Jimmy's exceptional understanding of his condition sufficient to allow Jimmy's refusal to stand?

The general rule of competence is that children are presumed incompetent to make legally binding decisions until they reach the age of majority (usually age 18). Autonomy requires both the mental capacity to understand the long-term and subtle implications of choices faced as well as the disciplined ability to sacrifice short-term interests for one's overall well-being. Small children, for example, might refuse immunizations out of the fear of the pain of the needle stick, incapable of understanding their long-term interests. Others may be able to understand, but lack the will power to make the prudent decision.

Some minors, especially adolescents, may, however, be sufficiently autonomous that they can both understand the nature of the choices to be made and possess the power of the will to make the proper decisions. There is in the law a doctrine of the *mature minor* by which minors can be determined to be sufficiently mature to make their own medical decisions.[7]

Mr. Young, however, faces a somewhat different problem. Is he in a position to assess whether Jimmy Scott is sufficiently mature to make a life-and-death decision on his own without the review of the courts? If Mr. Young is wrong in deciding about Jimmy's capacity, the result could be a death that perhaps should have been avoided. On the other hand, the alternative might be forcing the boy and his family to go through a burdensome court review.

There is another problem. Suppose that Jimmy, acting in a way that Mr. Young considers mature, reaches a decision that his parents reject. Suppose, for example, that Jimmy decides to refuse the treatment, while his parents insist that it be provided. If Jimmy is sufficiently mature to be able to make a substantially autonomous decision, do his parents have any right to overrule him? If the moral goal is preserving autonomy, then does the minor deemed mature have as much authority to make the decision on his own against his parent's wishes as he does to make it on his own when his parents concur?

2. Autonomy and the Mentally Impaired Adult

In some cases, determination of whether the patient is sufficiently autonomous to make his or her own decisions involves not children, but mentally impaired adults. These impairments may be the result of mental retardation or mental illness. In either case, the problem is how to determine whether the patient is sufficiently autonomous to make his or her own choices.

CASE 26: May a Suicidal Patient Refuse a Gastrostomy?

Herb Harrison was a 26-year-old white man. He was admitted with a self-inflicted gunshot wound to the soft palate in an attempt to commit suicide. He tested positive for marijuana and alcohol. At admission, the patient was 5′8″ and weighed 145 pounds. An attempt was made to remove the bullet and to close a fistula at the base of the brain. Both procedures were unsuccessful.

Ruth Reimer, the dietitian on call, started the patient on peripheral parenteral nutrition (PPN). Then half-strength Iso Cal @ 50 cc/hour was initiated through nasogastric (NG) tube. The patient couldn't tolerate by mouth feeding (P.O.); he aspirated any time by mouth feeding was initiated. As a result, an attempt was made to put in permanent gastrostomy, but the patient refused. Was the patient sufficiently autonomous to refuse the gastrostomy?

Herb Harrison is an adult who, under normal circumstances, has the moral and legal right to refuse medical treatments proposed for his own good. It seems highly debatable, however, whether his judgment about his own welfare is right in this case. He has decided he would be better off dead even before the critical medical problems from the self-inflicted gunshot wound emerged. Since he did not die from the gunshot, he apparently believes his best interest will now be served if he refuses a gastrostomy. Assuming that he needs the gastrostomy to live, he is, in effect, deciding that he still would be better off dead. His future life prospect is so bleak, so negative on balance, that the zero of death seems desirable.

In Chapter 3 we saw that there is room for conflict over what counts as the good for a patient. We saw that there were times when a patient's medical good—measured in part by future life expectancy—might conflict with his good overall, where the quality of life might conflict with the quantity of it.

In these circumstances Ruth Reimer and other members of the health care team know very little about the exact causes of Mr. Harrison's suicide attempt and how accurately he can estimate his long-term best interest. If you were Ruth Reimer, would you work on the assumption that continued life was in Mr. Harrison's interest?

It is possible that Ms. Reimer could reach the conclusion that his suicide was caused by an underlying treatable depression and that the gastrostomy would provide the opportunity for that therapy. Assuming that she concluded that continued life was in his interest, should Mr. Harrison still have the moral right, grounded in autonomy, to make his own choice to end his life (even if doing so is contrary to his own interest)?

Some patients are mentally so incapable of making rational decisions that they should have decision-making authority taken from them. Small children, the comatose, and the severely retarded seem clear examples. Others are capable of expressing some clear choice, but unable to reason through all the implications of their choice. This might be because of temporary insanity or severe constraints on knowledge. Is the fact that someone is suicidal automatic evidence that he or she lacks the ability to understand the choice they are making? Is there any evidence that Mr. Harrison lacks that capacity?

What should Ms. Reimer do if she believes that Mr. Harrison has that capacity? What should she do if she believes that he lacks it? Some philosophers distinguish between hard and soft paternalism.[8] Paternalism is hard if it involves overriding the decision of another on the grounds the choice is not in the decision maker's best interest *even though the decision maker is a substantially autonomous person*. Paternalism is soft if it involves overriding another long enough to determine whether the individual is acting in a substantially autonomous fashion. If Ms. Reimer intervenes in this case, is she manifesting strong or weak paternalism and why?

EXTERNAL CONSTRAINTS ON AUTONOMY

Persons may be substantially autonomous in the sense that they have the neurological and mental capacity as well as adequate knowledge, but still be constrained for specific choices by external forces. Persons in special institutions, sometimes called "total" institutions, such as prisons, boarding schools, or the military, may be subject to forces that exert substantial control on their choices. Persons may also be under the threat of physical force.

One interesting problem in this area is whether persons have their autonomy violated when they are pressured by "irresistibly attractive offers." For example, if an imprisoned sexual offender is offered release if, and only if, he agrees to an implant of a long-acting hormone that is expected to control his sexual aggression, is such a person able to choose autonomously to accept or reject the offer? If not, is it because the offer is made while he is in prison, or is it because the option seems so attractive compared to the alternative? Ethical problems of respect for autonomy can be created by the external forces such as these. The following case illustrates the problem.

CASE 27: External Constraints on Autonomy

Wanda Evans has just accepted a new position as assistant professor of medical technology at West Coast University. She will be responsible for teaching junior- and senior-level courses in hematology, a junior immunology course, and a senior clinical correlation seminar. Her responsibilities include didactic instruction in the classroom and student laboratory, coordination of the students' clinical experiences in hematology, advising a portion of the students in the major, maintaining an active research program, and service to the university and community.

West Coast University is a comprehensive university with 14 schools and colleges located in a rural environment. The medical technology program is administratively housed in the School of Human Services with programs in Social Work, Health Administration, Speech and Hearing, and Occupational Therapy. The university does not own a hospital, but has formal affiliation agreements with a community hospital 12 miles from the campus.

During her orientation, Ms. Evans learned from her colleagues that the major source of normal laboratory specimens for student instruction was the students themselves. Students perform venipunctures and capillary punctures on their classmates to obtain the necessary samples for analysis in their laboratory classes.

All students in the medical technology program sign a waiver giving the university permission to use their blood and body fluids for educational purposes. Further, they give written permission for venipunctures as needed.

When she questioned the practice of using student specimens as the primary source of laboratory materials, Ms. Evans was told that the students had the ability to refuse to participate. The other faculty viewed the students participation as voluntary. In their experience, no student had ever refused to sign the waiver form and/or permission slip.

Ms. Evans was not reassured by her colleagues' response. She felt uncomfortable about the issue of confidentiality of individual results, and she was especially concerned about the true level of voluntariness in the process. Are the students truly free to refuse? Has the students' autonomy been reduced by pressure from peers and fear of failure? Is there an implied threat from the faculty in the process? Ms. Evans was uncertain if it was ethical for her to adopt this same practice for her immunology and hematology classes.

The fact that the students in this case are college students implies that they have the maturity and intellectual capacity to understand the nature of the choice being presented if they are asked to volunteer to provide their own blood samples. As was noted earlier, in most jurisdictions the age of majority is 18. That is the age at which research subjects would be permitted to volunteer to be in a research project without their parents' permission. We can assume that, since these students are in college in junior- and senior-level courses, they are well above the normal age at which they can give consent for such activities.

Furthermore, the risks of providing the blood through venipunctures and capillary punctures seem minimal. The fact that fellow students are performing the procedures increases the risks somewhat. Does it increase the risks to an unreasonable level? Would an institutional review board have any objection to asking these students to give blood for research outside the educational setting if the students were told the one drawing the blood was a student?

Now, assuming that the risks are well within bounds, what is the relevance of the fact that this is being considered within an educational setting in which the student's evaluation depends on the impression he or she makes on the instructor? In what sense, if any, are these students "coerced" into consenting? If they were told that they could freely choose to give the blood and pass the course or refuse to give and fail the course, in what way, if any, is their response coerced?

Many universities have reached the conclusion that it is unethically coercive for psychology professors to insist that their students "volunteer" for research projects as part of their instruction in psychology. Is the request to consent to give blood for educational purposes the same thing?

Medical technologists must somehow learn to draw blood and must have a source of blood to practice laboratory analysis. If Ms. Evans is prohibited ethically from asking her students to practice on each other and generate their own blood for practice, where should this experience come from? If people who were not students were offered sufficient money to volunteer to give blood and be subjects of practice needle sticks by students, would their agreement be more or less coerced than if the students are asked? If only low-income persons "volunteer," are they as coerced by their economic circumstances as the students are by their desire for an education?

Suppose the school decides to ask prisoners at a local facility to provide the blood samples and practice for the students. If they can be expected to gain the respect of the warden for volunteering and have nothing else to do to occupy their time, are they coerced by external constraints into offering to participate? If any of these external constraints makes the request for volunteering unethical, what makes it unethical? Is lack of choice per se unacceptable? Does the fact that the offer (a degree if you consent) is so attractive in comparison with the alternatives make the offer unacceptable? When is it that external forces make a personal choice nonautonomous?

OVERRIDING THE CHOICES OF AUTONOMOUS PERSONS

Up to this point, this chapter has dealt with persons whose autonomy is debated, either because of inherent lack of the internal capacity to make substantially autonomous choices or because of external constraints that could make specific choices nonautonomous. Some persons, however, are substantially autonomous. They possess both the internal capacity to make choices according to their life plan and are in an environment that offers them reasonable freedom to choose without external constraints. Still the choice they make may seem to be very foolish. It may seem to offer risks of harms that far exceed any benefits that could be gained. Assuming, for purposes of discussion, that a person is substantially autonomous, is there ever a time when it is ethically justified to constrain his or her actions for the individual's own good or does the principle of autonomy always win out, requiring that the autonomous individual's own choices be respected insofar as it is only that individual whose interests are jeopardized?

CASE 28: Overriding Autonomy

Donald Taylor is a 48-year-old male who has had three previous attacks of kidney stones. Each of those times, he had an Intravenous Pylogram (IVP) examination, which consists of taking a series of timed x-rays with a contrast medium. The contrast medium consists largely of iodine. In each of the previous three examinations, Mr. Taylor has not had any difficulty with the contrast medium even though it can produce dangerous side effects including death.

Now, Mr. Taylor has had a new kidney stone attack, which results in his once again being sent to the Radiography Department for an IVP. On each occasion, Tyronne Downs has been the technologist who has taken Mr. Taylor's x-rays. This fourth time, the physician in the department provides a more detailed statement of the possible complications to Mr. Taylor. Death is indicated as being a possible outcome of the examination.

At first, Mr. Taylor indicates that he will go through with the procedure, but then expresses some grave doubts to Mr. Downs. Mr. Taylor asks Mr. Downs to say something to the physician. Mr. Downs, knowing that Mr. Taylor has not had a problem in the past, does not convey Mr. Taylor's extreme degree of concern to the physician who is supposed to administer the contrast medium. He is worried that if Mr. Taylor hears more about possible terrible outcomes, even if the risk is extremely remote, he will irrationally refuse the procedure. He realizes that Mr. Taylor is in extreme pain and feels it would be better for him to get on with the IVP as soon as possible without long, drawn out discussion of the remote side effects. When the time comes for the procedure, Mr. Taylor assumes that his concern has been expressed. He does not want to appear to be challenging the authority of the physician and does not want to consume his time, so he says nothing further. The IVP goes forward with the physician administering the contrast medium, unaware of the patient's concern.

There is every reason to assume that Mr. Taylor has the mental capacity to understand and discuss the nature of the risks of the IVP. When the technologist, Mr. Downs, learns of the patient's reservations, he, in effect, realizes that the patient is not giving a completely autonomous consent to participate in the procedure. He envisions that Mr. Taylor might refuse the procedure even though it has not been a problem in the past and, presumably, the physician believes that the risk is worth it.

If Mr. Downs is convinced that the IVP is in the patient's interest and is worth the risk, should he go ahead without speaking out? If he suspects the patient would resist the procedure if he were given more of an opportunity to think through the risks, is that a sufficient reason to minimize the discussion?

Mr. Taylor has, in this case, actually been informed of the risks, even the risk of death. Does that mean that, since he has been informed, he is acting autonomously? What can we make of the fact that Mr. Taylor seemed very concerned and yet he went ahead with the procedure even though the technologist did not raise the issue with the physician? Does that mean that the patient was acting autonomously?

Mr. Downs has been involved in this very procedure with the same patient on three previous occasions (when the patient was unaware of the small risk of death). Was Mr. Taylor acting autonomously when he had the procedure on the previous occasions? What would it take for Mr. Taylor to act autonomously in this case? Is it Mr. Downs' job to see that he be given the chance to act autonomously?

Other examples of cases in which allied health professionals may consider whether it is morally acceptable to violate the autonomy of a patient arise when the medical well-being of the patient appears to conflict with his or her religious commitments. Christian Scientists, Jehovah's Witnesses, and members of other religious groups hold views that proscribe certain medical interventions even though it is recognized by most people in the society that these interventions will help save lives. Another point of conflict arises over dietary laws of Judaism. In the following case a similar problem arises with a Muslim patient.

CASE 29: Tricked into a Good Diet

Mr. M.N. was a 78-year-old male hospitalized at County Medical Center with renal failure for which he receives dialysis three times per week. He was a Type II diabetic with anemia secondary to renal insufficiency. He was admitted in May 1989 because of an arrhythmia and was placed on a renal diet. He was not eating hospital meat (beef, pork, lamb, and poultry) because of his religious beliefs. The patient was a Muslim.

The Medical Center food service department does not serve "hallal meat," which is prepared through a special slaughtering process like kosher meat. (Muslims do not eat kosher meat, although the process of slaughtering is the same.) At the hospital he was eating like a vegetarian. The physician restricted his egg intake to two per week because of his heart condition, and he did not like Eggbeaters®. Milk was restricted in his diet secondary to his elevated phosphorous level in the blood.

It was hard to provide adequate high-biological-value protein, and while his appetite was poor, the patient refused nutritional supplements. Parenteral feeding was not appropriate.

James Kelly, the dietitian, found two ways to make him eat hospital food.

1. Make him believe the hospital provides hallal meat and what he eats is hallal.
2. Refer to Islam (with which, admittedly, Mr. Kelly was not very familiar); offer reasons to show him that, according to his religion, he should eat nonhallal meat in emergency situations like this one. He had some vague knowledge this was, in fact, consistent with Muslim belief as it is with Judaism.

Mr. Kelly seems convinced that it is important to Mr. N's welfare to get him to eat more protein. Assuming that is correct, and that there was no other way to get him to consume enough protein, is it morally justified to trick him into believing that he is eating hallal meat? The principle of autonomy holds that actions are improper insofar as they prevent a person from acting according to his own life plan. Is that what Mr. Kelly would be doing if he said the meat was hallal? If so, is the violation of his autonomy justified in an extreme case such as this?

What about the second alternative? It is true that kosher diet laws may be broken, in fact must be broken, to save a life.[9] Muslim ethics is similar, but Mr. Kelly apparently is not really sure.[10] Would it be ethical to take advantage of his vague knowledge to get Mr. N to eat or should he pursue a more reliable statement of Muslim beliefs first? Are there other options open to Mr. Kelly? Would it be better to encourage family members to bring properly prepared food from home (even if the nutritional value was less clearly understood by Mr. Kelly)? Should he try to bring someone to the hospital who is a teacher of Islam who could clarify the exact nature of the dietary prohibition? If these fail, is the lie to try to save a life justified?

PROVIDER AUTONOMY

Thus far the issues raised by the cases in this chapter have focused on client autonomy—whether the client has the internal capacity for autonomous choices and whether the client is sufficiently free from external constraints—and on whether the client should be free to make choices that seem to the health care provider to be unwise.

Patients and clients are not the only ones who raise questions about the moral right to act autonomously. Health care providers are also moral agents capable of making substantially autonomous choices. The moral principle of autonomy holds that, insofar as choices affect only the one making the choices, persons should be free to make their own choices according to their own life plans, even if those choices do not maximize their welfare. The principle holds even more powerfully when it appears that the choices do serve the decision maker's interests. This is the moral basis of the position expressed by many professional organizations that health care providers have the moral right to determine which clients they shall serve and under what circumstances.

Nevertheless, it is widely recognized that health care professionals have certain duties to serve their patients or clients. Those duties are seen as either inherent in the role of being a health professional or as part of a "social contract" that is part of the licensure of health professionals. This case illustrates how the autonomy of the health care provider can generate moral controversy.

CASE 30: Refusing a Diabetic Diet

A 50-year-old Oriental female, Sun Yong Chen, was admitted with diabetic ulcer on her left heel. The patient is 5′ 11½″ tall and weighs 236 pounds. The norm is 158 pounds on a 2,000-calorie American Dietetic Association diet. Patient Daily Energy Expenditure 1416, Total Energy Expenditure 1699-1841. A 1,400-calorie diet was recommended for weight reduction. The patient was also advised to attend classes for diabetics offered in the hospital. The patient refused the 1,400-calorie diet and persuaded the physician to order 2,000 calories. The patient also refused the standard saline distributions. Instead, she was consuming a total of 10 oz. of meat and 70 grams of fat each day. The patient was educated on the principles of diabetic diet, but she continued to insist on doing things her way. Finally, the dietitian, Rosie Maynard, has to give in to patient demands.

Mrs. Chen apparently understands the risks and benefits of her diet. What are those risks and benefits? How should Ms. Maynard, the dietitian, determine the risks and benefits of not being on the diabetic diet? Is she capable of determining how uncomfortable Mrs. Chen is following the diet and how bad it is for her if she does not follow it?

Suppose that Ms. Maynard really can determine whether the risks of abandoning the diet are worth it from Mrs. Chen's point of view, and she determines that they are not. Perhaps Mrs. Chen herself acknowledges she would be better off in the long run following the diet and would like to follow it. Would that justify refusing to give in to Mrs. Chen's demands for a less restrictive fare? If acting autonomously is bad for the patient, does that justify a health professional's decision to restrict autonomy?

Ms. Maynard apparently concludes that she does not have the moral right (or legal right) to coerce Mrs. Chen into the diet she recommends. She appears to believe that she must give in to Mrs. Chen's demands. But if Mrs. Chen has a moral right not to accept Ms. Maynard's recommendation because she is an autonomous agent, does Ms. Maynard also have the moral right in such a case to sever the relationship and refuse to be part of Mrs. Chen's dangerous life-style? She is also an autonomous agent. Does that give her the right to choose to continue professional relations on whatever basis she chooses including insisting that she will only take patients who are at least minimally cooperative?

Generally, autonomous persons have no obligation to remain in relations that violate their sense of what is proper. Are health professionals any different? When they accept a position as the dietitian for the ward in the hospital, are they committing themselves to trying to assist all patients no matter how they eat, or do they have the right to act autonomously and withdraw from the case?

If Ms. Maynard decides to withdraw from Mrs. Chen's case, what obligation, if any, does she have to Mrs. Chen? When physicians withdraw from cases on grounds of conscience, they usually arrange for someone else to take over the case. If Ms. Maynard is the only one on the ward, what arrangement should she make? What arrangement could she make?

ENDNOTES

1. For good discussions of the principle of autonomy and related concepts, see Joel Feinberg, "Legal Paternalism," in his *Rights, Justice, and the Bounds of Liberty: Essays in Social Philosophy* (Princeton, NJ: Princeton University Press, 1980), pp. 110-129; Gerald Dworkin, "Moral Autonomy," in *Morals, Science, and Society*, eds. H. Tristram Engelhardt and Daniel Callahan (Hastings-on-Hudson, NY: The Hastings Center, 1978), pp. 156-171; and Tom L. Beauchamp and James F. Childress, eds., *Principles of Biomedical Ethics*, 4th ed. (New York: Oxford University Press, 1994), pp. 120-188.
2. See the extended discussion of this approach in The Hastings Center, *Guidelines on the Termination of Life-Sustaining Treatment and the Care of the Dying* (Briarcliff Manor, NY: The Hastings Center, 1987), pp. 20-29.
3. John Stuart Mill, *On Liberty* (New York: Liberal Arts Press, 1956).
4. American Occupational Therapists Association, *Occupational Therapy Code of Ethics*, 1994.
5. Judith Areen, "The Legal Status of Consent Obtained from Families of Adult Patients to Withhold or Withdraw Treatment," *Journal of the American Medical Association*, Vol. 258, no. 2 (July 10, 1987), pp. 229-235; Robert M. Veatch,

"Limits of Guardian Treatment Refusal: A Reasonableness Standard," *American Journal of Law and Medicine*, Vol. 9, no. 4 (Winter 1984), pp. 427-468.

6. Paul S. Appelbaum, Charles W. Lidz, and Alan Meisel, *Informed Consent: Legal Theory and Clinical Practice* (New York: Oxford University Press, 1987), pp. 66-69.
7. Angela R. Holder, "Minors' Rights to Consent to Medical Care," *Journal of the American Medical Association*, Vol. 257, no. 24 (June 26, 1987), pp. 3400-3402.
8. Joel Feinberg, *Harm to Self: The Moral Limits of the Criminal Law*, Vol. 3 (New York: Oxford University Press, 1986), p. 12.
9. Fred Rosner and J. David Bleich, eds., *Jewish Bioethics* (New York: Sanhedrin Press, 1979), p. 19; Abraham S. Abraham, *Medical Halachah for Everyone* (Jerusalem: Feldheim, 1984), pp. 9-13.
10. A. Yusuf Ali, ed., *The Holy Quran* (Chicago: Kazi, 1983), S. II. 173, pp. 67-68, S. V. 3, pp. 239-240; Fazlur Rahman, *Health and Medicine in the Islamic Tradition: Change and Identity* (New York: Crossroad, 1987), pp. 50-54.

CHAPTER 6

Veracity

DEALING HONESTLY WITH CLIENTS

In the previous chapter health providers were in positions in which they had to choose between doing what they thought was best for clients and respecting the client's autonomy. The moral principle of autonomy was in conflict with the principle of beneficence. We saw that some people held that respect for autonomy can take precedence over doing good for the patient.

The respect for autonomy is an element of a more general moral concept of respect for persons. Respect for persons, according to this view, sometimes requires moral choices that do not maximize the client's well-being.

Another element of respect for persons deals with honest disclosure. Traditional ethics holds that it is simply wrong morally to lie to people, even if it is expedient to do so, even if greater good will come from the lie. According to this view, lying to people is morally wrong in that it shows lack of respect for them. Expressed as a moral principle, holders of this view claim that veracity or honesty or truth-telling is a moral requirement. The principle conveys that dishonesty in actions or practices is an element of actions that makes them wrong. As with justice and autonomy, there may also be other dimensions of these actions that tend toward making them right. For example, the fact that a lie produces good results would tend to make it right. However, holders of this view maintain that, nevertheless, the lie itself is an element that makes the action wrong. It is, according to this approach, *prima facie* wrong, that is, wrong insofar as the lying dimension is considered.

It is striking that even though many common moral systems treat lying as wrong in and of itself, traditional health care ethics has not. Thus, the Hippocratic Oath does not require that physicians deal honestly with patients. Similarly, some of the codes of allied health professional groups do not explicitly require honesty in dealing with patients. Many professional medical ethics have, in fact, maintained that it is right for a physician to lie to a patient when doing so will spare the patient agony. In this sense professional medical ethics has focused on the consequences of actions, not on any inherent moral elements whether they be respecting autonomy or telling the truth.

Ethics that focus on consequences, such as the Hippocratic Oath, accept lies when they produce benefit. Classical utilitarian ethics assesses the acceptability of a lie based on the total consequences. It considers the benefits and harms for all parties.[1] By contrast, traditional health professional ethics looks only to the consequences for the patient.[2] The cases in this chapter present situations in which allied health professionals believe that they can benefit their clients by lying or at least withholding the truth.

While ethics that focus on consequences try to determine whether a lie will produce benefit, the ethics that emphasize nonconsequentialist elements such as respect for persons, hold that there is something simply wrong about lying. Immanuel Kant the eighteenth-century philosopher, is most closely identified with this view.[3] Twentieth-century thinkers have agreed.[4] While physicians traditionally accepted the legitimacy of lying to patients in order to protect them,[5] more recent developments suggest that physicians are changing, perhaps giving greater emphasis to the patient's right to the truth.[6]

The allied health professions present different views about truth-telling in their codes. The code of the American Dietetic Association commits its members to honesty, integrity, and fairness.[7] The American Occupational Therapy Association commits its members to the view that "Occupational therapy personnel shall fully inform the service recipients of the nature, risks, and potential outcomes of treatment." Moreover, they shall inform subjects involved in research activities of the potential risks and outcome of those activities.[8] Physical therapists, according to their code, are committed to "provide accurate information to the consumer about the profession and about those services they provide."[9]

By contrast, some of the codes are silent about any duty to speak truthfully to patients just as the older versions of the American Medical Association's *Principle of Ethics* were.[10] For example, the American Academy of Physician Assistants code pledges the physician assistant to work for the welfare of patients, but does not specifically require him or her to deal honestly with them.[11] Since the major justification for failing to be honest with patients is the fear that certain information could upset or harm a patient, those who subscribe to traditional health care ethics of the Hippocratic tradition would deduce that the duty to serve the patient's welfare justifies certain dishonesties with patients. The American Society of Radiologic Technologists is unique in committing the radiology technologist to "obtain pertinent information for the physician to aid in the diagnosis and treatment management of the patient" while not mentioning honesty in dealing with patients.[12] Still other codes, commit simultaneously to promoting the best interests of the patient and the right of the patient to be informed, leaving the question of this chapter: What should be done when the allied health professional believes that it is in the patient's best interest to withhold the truth?[13]

The cases in this chapter will begin with the special problem of what clients should be told when the health care provider himself or herself is not yet sure what the facts are. Then a series of cases involving the problem of lying to patients to benefit them will be explored followed by cases in which the health provider considers lying to the patient to benefit others. The chapter will then take up two special situations involving veracity—cases in which first the patient and then the patient's family asks not to be told. Finally, a case explores disclosure to patients who ask to see their medical record.

THE CONDITION OF DOUBT

Before discussing the ethics of disclosure, it is important to get some sense of exactly what it is that might be disclosed. In health care a problem arises frequently that can be referred to as the "condition of doubt." It arises when the health care provider is in real doubt about what the facts are.

The confusion may be in regard to a diagnosis about which the health care professional has only a preliminary suspicion. The doubt may arise when innovative therapies are contemplated and the health care provider is not clear about what the effects of the treatment will be. He or she may not even know whether the doubt is from personal ignorance of the current literature or because even the leading authorities are unclear.

In allied health the condition of doubt may arise because the health care provider has only limited knowledge and knows that someone else on the health care team is better informed. In these cases even one who is in principle militantly committed to dealing honestly with the patient may not know exactly what should be said. The first case in this chapter raises this problem.

CASE 31: Communicating Preliminary Research Data

Medical researchers at Cooke University hypothesized that a newly developed antibiotic, if taken during pregnancy, was an effective drug for reducing infant mortality rates. Few side effects have been associated with the drug, but its effect on the developing fetus has not been determined. They have received backing from the drug manufacturer to do a pilot study. If the research hypothesis is proven, the manufacturing company stands the chance to make a hefty profit, and the university will likely be awarded major contracts to implement projects in various countries.

Realizing the "red tape" and long waiting period to get such a pilot project approved in the United States, a poor and developing country with high infant mortality rates was selected and approved by the funder of the study. Researchers rationalize that if expectant mothers in this country have lowered rates of infection, infant mortality rates will be decreased, and this will work toward improving the economy.

A study sample of 2,000 expectant mothers was selected and divided into two groups. Each mother was given a $50.00 per week stipend incentive. Group I was given one antibiotic capsule per day; Group II was given a sugar placebo capsule per day. Three months into the study, 10 mothers in Group I had suffered miscarriages, compared to 6 in Group II. After careful statistical analysis, it was determined that the miscarriage rate, although slightly higher in Group I, was not statistically significant. The decision was made to continue the study.

Several group participants are now worried that they may lose their babies and wonder if they should continue in the study. They are reassured by the PA, Tom Staley, who implements the research protocols and are told, "I don't think you have anything to worry about. All the studies conducted so far show no harmful effects on the developing babies."

If a study had been completed and had shown at a high level of statistical significance that the patients taking the experimental drug had two-thirds higher mortality rate, it seems unlikely that the physician's assistant would have any difficulty figuring out what the patients should be told. Mr. Staley would feel morally obliged to tell the patients about the mortality risk. In fact, the drug surely would be banned from the market, at least in the United States.

But Mr. Staley's situation is quite different. Consider the truthful statements that he might have said about the study. He could have said, "There has never been any statistically significant evidence that the drug does any harm." Or he could have said, "The study is at such an early stage that there are no meaningful results yet available." Mr. Staley might have been entirely honest when he said, "I don't think you have anything to worry about."

Given that this study was being conducted in a developing country, he might have assumed that the subjects would not have understood the references to statistical significance. He might assume that the statement, "All of the studies conducted so far show no harmful effects on the developing babies," would mean about the same thing to these women as the statement, "There has never been any statistically significant evidence that the drug does any harm." On the other hand, he could also truthfully have said, "Even though the results are not yet statistically meaningful, so far there are more miscarriages for women taking the active experimental drug." If the earlier statements might be too reassuring, the latter might be too alarming.

The real problem here seems to be that Mr. Staley is confronted with a situation in which he really does not know what the effect of the drug will be. There are theoretical reasons to believe it might work. On the other hand, the data so far do not show the benefit; in fact they show a preliminary trend that, if it continues, will lead to the conclusion that the drug actually is doing harm. Mr. Staley is in a condition of doubt.

Many people who generally believe there is a moral duty to tell the truth also recognize that there are situations in which it is too early to tell what the truth is. If a respiratory care practitioner sees a patient who is a smoker and who had a persistent cough, laryngitis, and fever, the diagnosis of lung cancer may enter her mind, but that does not mean she should blurt out to the patient immediately that she may have lung cancer. Not only is there real doubt about the diagnosis at this point; there is also doubt that the therapist should be the one to raise the issue.

Mr. Staley must decide what counts as truthful, meaningful communication about the early results of the trial. It should be clear that no one wants what could be called the "full truth." There is an infinite number of things that could be said. No reasonable woman wants to know everything: the chemical structure of the drug, various theories of statistical testing, all the educational credentials of all the participants in the study. What is usually expected is information that is "reasonably meaningful." The problem in Mr. Staley's case is that it is not clear exactly what is reasonably meaningful. How should Mr. Staley respond to women who ask about the risks in an early phase of the study? What should a clinical care giver say when there is real doubt about what the truth is? Is it sufficient to say, "We don't know yet," or is there an obligation to spell out what is suspected or what concerns the clinician?

LYING IN ORDER TO BENEFIT

Resolving doubt about what the truth is is not all that is at stake in the ethics of truth-telling. In some cases the health care provider may know the truth, but fear that disclosing it to the patient will do the patient or someone else significant harm. Often it turns out that telling the truth is also beneficial, but the interesting moral cases are those in which honesty involves risk of hurting someone. In such cases, is there still a moral duty to tell the truth, or is it right to be honest only in those cases in which telling the truth is expected to be beneficial? The following cases are ones in which someone is worried about hurting someone by being honest.

1. Protecting the Patient by Lying

Often it is the patient who could be injured—psychologically or physically—if the health care provider is completely honest. Among the issues presented in the following case are (1) is avoiding the truth any different morally than telling an outright lie, (2) how can the allied health professional know what the consequences will be, (3) can the problem be avoided by referring the patient to the physician for disclosure, and (4) what is the nature of the duty to be honest?

CASE 32: Lying About the Cancer Evidence

Elise Jackson is a medical technologist who has recently assumed responsibility as supervisor of phlebotomy services at her hospital. In both her personal and professional life, she has always believed deeply that her integrity is measured by her honesty with other people. She feels strongly about telling the truth to patients because she respects their autonomy and insists that they have a "right-to-know" in order to make appropriate decisions.

During a workshop on medicolegal issues, the risk manager noted that it was not the responsibility of the phlebotomist to inform the patient of the tests to be performed on the samples they obtained. This view was contradictory to the basic beliefs of the supervisor.

Surely the institution could not sanction lying to patients. If direct questions were posed by patients, they had a right to a response if the care giver had the information. Providing no response, referring the question, or lying were all unprofessional and unethical in Ms. Jackson's mind.

The experienced phlebotomy staff concurred with the risk manager that they did not always feel a responsibility to answer truthfully. They made judgments about the impact of their answers; depending upon how well they knew the patient, what other information the patient had, the patient's prognosis and service, they would temporize or even lie. It was not always in the patient's best interest to tell the truth. They suggested that Ms. Jackson spend a two-week period functioning as a staff phlebotomist so that she might gain an appreciation for this situation.

Following her staff's advice, Ms. Jackson scheduled herself for two weeks of morning rounds on the medical-surgical wing. She found the experience to be very rewarding as she enjoyed the interaction with the patients and other health professionals. For the first week and a half, she was not presented with any situations in which she was not able to be completely honest. However, that changed.

A 47-year-old male was admitted to her floor as a follow-up of surgery for colorectal cancer six months earlier. He informed her on the first day of his hospital stay that he was greatly concerned about a recurrence of the cancer. He was adamant in his belief that it was better to die then, while he was feeling relatively well, than to live another year and suffer. He stated that he would take his own life if he learned that there was more cancer present in his bowel.

One of the tests performed on admission was a caranoembryonic antigen (CEA). Because of the patient's intense commentary, Ms. Jackson looked through the laboratory results and learned that his CEA level was elevated, which presented strong evidence for residual cancer. On his second hospital day, further lab studies were ordered, which required Ms. Jackson to perform a venipuncture. At that time she was asked if all the preceding day's tests were normal.

Ms. Jackson was certain that this patient would attempt to end his life if he learned that he probably had cancer, yet she did not want to compromise her own integrity by not telling the truth. The consequences of either action were unpleasant for her. What was the best course to follow?

First, consider the distinction often drawn between lying and failing to tell the truth. Were she to say that the CEA was negative, she would not only be telling a lie, she would probably be found out. The physician would quite possibly discuss the accurate findings. Saying the test is negative is typical of a lie that, in the end, would have bad consequences.

What, however, if she dishonestly said she did not know the results of the test? That would be just as much of a lie, but it is much less likely she would be found out. What are the likely consequences of that lie?

If Ms. Jackson believes that both she and the patient would be better off telling an outright lie in cases when everyone benefits and she is not likely to get caught, what moral reason would there be not to tell the lie? Some, such as Kantians, respond at this point that there is just something unethical about telling such lies—even when everyone is better off for the lie being told. People who hold such a view believe that there is a moral principle that it is wrong to lie regardless of the consequences. This principle, sometimes called the principle of veracity, identifies all knowingly wrongful statements as unethical, at least in regard to the lie.

But what if Ms. Jackson simply refuses to say anything one way or another? Or what if she says something like, "I cannot discuss the results of the test with you. You will need to speak to your physician about that." Now she would not be lying; she simply would be withholding the truth. Does that also violate the principle of veracity?

It seems clear that, even if all outright dishonest statements are morally wrong, no one has a moral duty to say everything she knows about other people. At the same time health professionals have a duty to make sure patients are adequately informed so that they can make autonomous choices about the treatment options. Informed consent requires that patients get relevant information truthfully. This suggests that health professionals have an obligation to disclose relevant information, even if ordinary citizens do not always have such obligations.

In this case, Ms. Jackson envisions what she takes to be horrible consequences if her patient knows the result of the tests. It seems hard to deny that the test results are relevant to the patient's situation. Are the predicted consequences enough to justify not revealing the results? Suppose Ms. Jackson knows the patient's attending physician and is aware that he follows a normal practice of not disclosing cancer diagnostic information to his patients. Does that make it more imperative for Ms. Jackson to see that the patient is informed (on the grounds that she is the only one who will tell), or does that make it her duty to cooperate with the physician's strategy and refrain from disclosing?

2. Protecting the Welfare of Others

In the previous case a health care provider contemplated lying or withholding the truth because she thought it would be better for the patient not to know. Sometimes it is not the patient but someone else—a colleague or friend—whose welfare could be protected if the truth were withheld. In the following case, a lab technician is asked to protect a nurse who made an innocent and apparently harmless mistake.

CASE 33: Discovering a Mistaken Identity

Benita Johnson is a lab technician in the busy private practice of a group of allergists. She is responsible for maintaining the serums for the hundreds of patients who come routinely to the office for injections. On Monday, March 21, a request came from part-time nurse, Sandra Critton, for serum for Theodora Williams. Ms. Johnson knew Theodora, a young patient who normally went by the name Winnie, but she did not actually see her in the office. She supplied the nurse with the serum for the injection.

The next day Ms. Johnson was surprised to receive another request for serum for Winnie Williams, this time from another part-time nurse who had not worked the previous day. Since Ms. Williams should not be coming so frequently, Ms. Johnson decided to confirm that Ms. Williams was really in the office. She discovered that she was.

Upon investigation she discovered that the previous patient was actually Theodora Wilson. The ID numbers of the two patients had been confused on the order forms. Theodora Wilson, it was clear, had actually received Winnie Williams' serum. The error was made by the nurse who was on duty on Monday. Although there was some possibility of injury, by the time the error was discovered, it was clear that no real harm had been done. There was an ample supply of serum for both patients. Ms. Wilson was to be charged $6.00 for the injection.

Sandra Critton, the nurse who was responsible for the error, was terribly distressed. She did not realize that the office was seeing two patients with such similar names. She insisted she would be much more careful in the future and that such a thing would never happen again. She pleaded with Ms. Johnson not to tell Dr. Roberts, the physician in charge.

Assuming that Ms. Johnson believes no harm was actually done to the patients other than the cost of the erroneous injection, should Ms. Johnson comply with the nurse's request to ignore the mistake? Should she tell Dr. Roberts? What should she do if, after telling Dr. Roberts, he makes it clear that Ms. Wilson will not be told of the error and that she will be charged for erroneous injection? Would it make any difference if there were no charge for the injection?

A potentially serious error has been made, but by the time it is discovered, it seems clear that no real harm has been done. If the patient receiving the erroneous injection is informed she could be refunded the undue charge, but not much else could be done for her. On the other hand, if she is told of the error, she could lose confidence in the physician and perhaps even stop seeing him.

The real benefit and harm in this case, however, are not to the patient; there are others who have much more to gain or lose. Clearly, Ms. Critton, the nurse who made the mistake, could be in trouble with her employer. She probably has learned her lesson and only could be harmed if the incident is reported. On the other hand, other patients have something at stake. They could benefit if a more rigorous set of controls were instituted as a result of reporting the incident.

Health care providers have traditionally been guided by the Hippocratic principle, which requires that they act only so as to benefit their patient. In this case the specific patient would not be helped significantly if the report were filed. Does that mean that Ms. Johnson need not report? Or do the interests of future patients become decisive in the decision? The *Code of Ethics* of the American Society for Medical Technology provides a somewhat more nuanced position than that of the Hippocratic tradition. It says, "Clinical laboratory professionals are accountable for the quality and integrity of the laboratory services they provide . . . as well as in striving to safeguard the patient from incompetent or illegal practice by others." But it also says, "Clinical laboratory professionals actively strive to establish cooperative and insightful working relationships with other health professionals, keeping in mind their primary objective to ensure a high standard of care for the patients they serve."[14] Does the reference to establishing cooperative and insightful working relationships with other health professionals justify keeping silence, or does the commitment to safeguarding patients require disclosure?

A utilitarian approach to this case would consider the possible benefits and harms to all parties, not just the patients. Should the nurse's well-being be considered relevant in calculating whether to disclose the incident?

Underlying this problem is the more general question of whether Ms. Johnson should handle her dilemma by calculating the consequences for any of the affected people. It seems that Dr. Roberts would want to know about such an incident, if only to make sure that the charts of the two patients are flagged with a caution. Does an employee owe information to the employer that the employer reasonably would want to know even if the disclosure will hurt a colleague? Assuming that Ms. Johnson and Sandra Critton could propose a more careful set of procedures to protect against mistaken identity of patients in the future from this incident without letting Dr. Roberts know that a mistake has already occurred, do they still owe him an account of the incident just to be honest with him?

Sometimes the conflict of interest between the patient and others may be more dramatic than in the previous case. Medical records administrators are in a position to see such conflicts when they have reason to believe that a chart has been altered to protect a physician or the hospital. In the following case, it was a physician who apparently lied in modifying a record, but it was the records administrator who faced the problem of whether to report the dishonesty.

CASE 34: Lying and the Welfare of Others

A patient was admitted to the hospital's Short Procedure Unit for the surgical removal of four impacted wisdom teeth. As required, a staff internist did a history and physical examination prior to admission. The dental surgeon removed the wisdom teeth and administered penicillin intermuscularly as a prophylactic. The patient had an immediate and violent reaction to the penicillin and, after prolonged and intensive care, recovered and was discharged.

On routine discharge analysis, the discharge clerk noted the record deficiencies (missing signatures on the operative report, history, and physical examination). Recognizing an interesting case, the clerk read much of the record; in reading the history, she noted that there was no mention of drug allergies, although the patient's previous record (which she had just retrieved to combine with the new admission) had a red stamp on the cover stating ALLERGIC TO PENICILLIN.

She placed the record with its deficiency notice into the incomplete record file for the dental surgeon and internist to sign. One week later, the record was again on her desk; on checking for the missing signatures, she was surprised to see that the patient history now included an additional sentence stating, "Patient denies any allergy to penicillin or other drugs." She then took the medical record and related this information to the medical records administrator, who has just received a telephone call from the hospital attorney to locate that patient's record for his review. Although the patient has made a full recovery, a malpractice suit has been initiated against the hospital, the internist, and the dental surgeon because of the penicillin reaction.

Let us assume that, if the record had been changed, the one who changed the record acted unethically. (Probably the action was illegal as well.) That is not a complicated moral conclusion. The real moral complexity here is not the initial changing of the record, but the duty of the medical records administrator who has secondhand information that the record has been changed. She has no reason to question the veracity of the discharge clerk; however, the allegation of tampering with the original documentation is a very serious one.

Should the medical records administrator's approach to the problem be one of calculating the consequences of reporting and not reporting, or should she hold to the principle of veracity insisting that she has a duty to make the record accurate even if the hospital and the medical staff are hurt by it?

Calculating the consequences of alternative courses of action is always a complicated business. From the patient's point of view, it is clear that the patient may have a great deal to gain economically if the report is filed. On the other hand, the patient has made a full recovery, and there is no medical benefit to the patient from making the report. In fact, the administrator may feel that the patient is only trying to take advantage of the accident to collect on a large malpractice suit.

While the Hippocratic ethic focuses only on the patient, a utilitarian ethic would factor in the interests of all parties affected, including not only the physicians and hospital, but the medical records administrator herself. In fact the 1985 revision of the *Code of Ethics* of the American Medical Record Association required that the medical record professional consider the interests of the patient (Code II and IX), the hospital or institution (Code IX), other professionals (Code I), and medical record professionals themselves (Codes I and X).[15] Is it acceptable, especially if the administrator believes the patient is trying to take unfair advantage of the situation, to suppress the truth in order to protect the physicians and hospital from harm? This concern seems to have been reflected in the *AMRA Code* that stated that medical record professionals, "act loyally within the bounds of professional standards toward his/her employer and the goals of the institution" (Code V). Is it acceptable for the administrator to consider that she could generate hostility from the physicians and the hospital administrator if she becomes a whistle blower? Is there a duty to get the truth exposed here regardless of the consequences, or is this a matter to be resolved by calculating the consequences for everyone involved and trying to do what will produce the best results? Such questions of duty appear to be of concern in the *AMRA Code of Ethics*, which states that the medical record administrator "refuses to participate in any improper preparation, alteration, or suppression of health reports or official minutes" (Code IX, 3). Many of these phrases were changed in the 1991 Code when the professional group was called the American Health Information Management Association.

SPECIAL CASES OF TRUTH-TELLING

Although the usual cases of truth-telling involve situations in which the health provider contemplates lying or withholding the truth in order to benefit the patient or benefit someone else, there are some special cases in which lies, deceptions, or withholdings of information may be justified. These include cases in which the patient or some member of the family requests that the truth be withheld.

1. Patients Who Don't Want to Be Told

Sometimes a patient is said to fear bad news. When being seen for a diagnosis of a potentially fatal disease, the patient himself or herself may explicitly ask the provider to avoid disclosing the bad news. A radiation therapist confronts the problem in the following case.

CASE 35: When the Patient Asks Not to Be Told

Julia Olson is a 68-year-old woman who has been diagnosed as having breast cancer. She is referred to the Radiation Therapy Technology Department of the local hospital for radiation after a lumpectomy of her right breast.

Sally Gray is the radiation therapist assigned to give Mrs. Olson her treatment. As a part of the treatment routine, it is the responsibility of the therapist to explain thoroughly all aspects of the treatment to the patient. When Sally Gray begins her explanation, Mrs. Olson indicates that she really doesn't want to hear a long explanation, she just wants to get the whole thing over.

Two additional attempts by Sally Gray result in the same outcome—that Mrs. Olson doesn't want to hear a lot of explanation about something that she really doesn't understand. Given this situation, should Sally Gray proceed to administer the radiation, or should she insist that Mrs. Olson not waive her right to information?

While earlier cases in this chapter involve health care providers who are inclined to withhold potentially traumatic information from patients, Sally Gray faces the opposite problem. She is not only willing to disclose the details of the radiation; she feels morally obliged to do so.

Mrs. Olson, however, appears less interested. She has a right to the truth, but does she have a duty to get it? The rights associated with autonomy and veracity, with consent and informing patients, are what can be called alienable rights. The one who has the right to information also may waive the right. Sometimes we might waive the right to information to which we are entitled because it seems too trivial. People leading busy lives cannot possibly stop to process all the details of the information to which they are entitled. But is it ethically acceptable to decline information about momentous, life-and-death events like treatment for cancer?

Assuming that Mrs. Olson continues to insist that she does not want to know the details, that is, that she waives her right to know, Ms. Gray has to decide whether to cooperate in the treatment of the uninformed patient. Presumably, health providers have the legal right to refuse any patient, but when allied health workers refuse, they do so within a health care system that may create psychological and social pressures. The real issue here, however, is whether there is any moral reason why Ms. Gray should refuse to cooperate.

2. Family Members Who Insist the Patient Not Be Told

A second special case involves a patient whose family insists the patient should not be told. Now it is the family member who is claiming the authority to waive the right to know. In some cases, such as the one that follows, it can be argued that the patient would be hurt, psychologically or physically, if he or she knew the threatening information. Nevertheless, the question persists whether there is anyone who has the authority to overturn the patient's claim on the information.

CASE 36: Ethics Consultation: The Case of Ms. R.

Ms. R. is a 25-year-old black female admitted to the hospital six months ago with pancreatitis. It was determined during that admission that Ms. R. has had a choledochal cyst as well. The cyst was removed, and she was given radiation therapy. Ms. R. has had several hospital admissions since her treatments with complaints of nausea and vomiting. She continued to be followed by her pediatrician, which is a separate issue of concern. Ms. R. is single and lives with her parents. She was employed full time prior to her first admission, but has not worked since that time. She describes her family as being "very close," with good relationships among all family members.

The issue centers on the fact that Ms. R.'s parents requested that she not be told that her cyst was malignant. Their rationale behind this request is Ms. R.'s previous statement that if she ever contracted cancer she did not want to know. Her parents felt that they were doing what was best by respecting their daughter's wishes.

Helen Westerman, the radiation therapist, believed that Ms. R. was an adult and had the right to know the truth regarding her illness in order to make her own decisions concerning her future. To be autonomous, the person must be free of external control and in control of his or her own affairs. This principle is being denied if her parents are allowed to control this situation.

Questions for Discussion

1. What are the rights of both the patient and her family?
2. What are the implications of each of these rights?
3. Which rights should carry the most weight?
4. What would be the best decision for the patient?

In some ways this case is like Case 35. Someone believes that the patient is better off not knowing. Yet in this case it is less clear that it is the patient who is waiving the right to be informed. Recently, in health care ethics patients have been given the right to appoint a surrogate (sometimes called a durable power of attorney) to make decisions when the patient is no longer capable. In some ways Ms. R. might be seen as having appointed her parents as surrogates. Is such surrogate decision making acceptable when the patient, like Ms. R., is still competent? Can a surrogate be appointed informally, or must the transfer of decision-making authority be done legally and in writing?

It is possible that Ms. R. did not really appoint her parents to make the decision about whether information should be held from her. If so, then the question is whether their concern about her welfare justifies withholding potentially meaningful information. Do parents, a spouse, or others concerned about the patient ever have the right to protect the patient from potentially traumatic information in cases that, unlike the previous case, do not involve the patient's waiver of the right to know?

A related issue worth discussing is how Ms. R.'s parents came to find out about the malignancy in the first place. The traditional ethics of confidentiality requires that information about a patient not be disclosed without the patient's permission. There is no evidence that Ms. R. gave the radiation therapist or anyone else permission to disclose her diagnosis to her parents before she found out about it. Does that constitute a violation of the ethics of confidentiality? Confidentiality will be discussed further in the cases of the next chapter.

THE RIGHT OF ACCESS TO MEDICAL RECORDS

Closely related to the ethics of truth-telling is the question of the right of access of a patient to his or her medical records. This is a problem for health information administrators, but also for all other health care providers. If the patient has the right to be told all that is potentially meaningful about his or her medical condition and treatment, does that also imply a right to see his or her medical records or at least to know what they contain?

CASE 37: The Right to Health Records

A registered nurse comes to the Medical Records Department of a rural health maintenance organization requesting copies of her now-deceased mother's prenatal care records prior to her own delivery. Her father is also deceased and the woman was an only child; she is the legally designated next of kin. She completes the appropriate authorization and prepays the standard fee for the copies. She leaves with the expectation that the copies will shortly be forthcoming.

She is concerned that her mother may have been treated with diethylstilbestrol (DES) during the pregnancy because of a recent questionable Pap smear and comments regarding the difficulty of the pregnancy made by an aunt at a recent family gathering. She wants to review her prenatal records herself to determine whether or not she is at increased risk of developing a malignancy. If her mother was treated with the drug, she plans to follow through with the recommended health care monitoring, but also intends to forward the records to an attorney for possible inclusion in a class action suit against the pharmaceutical company that made the drug. Although she was delivered by a general practitioner (now retired) in private practice, his patient records were transferred to the HMO when he and his partners became full-time staff of the HMO.

The medical records administrator locates the prenatal care records and forwards a routine notification to the physician about this request. Unexpectedly, the physician responds immediately by telephone that the record is not to be released. He is evasive when asked to document the reason for refusing the request in the record, but he says that he will write a letter to the daughter reassuring her that DES was not administered to her mother. The medical records administrator then reviews the prenatal records carefully. She finds no indication that DES was prescribed; however, she does find a notation in the prenatal history that the pregnancy was achieved via artificial insemination. No information is given about the sperm donor. The daughter has prepaid for copies of the records, and the medical records administrator must respond in some manner.

Although this case is more complicated than that of a patient who wants to see her own (postnatal) medical record, it might be argued that a prenatal record is not only the record of the mother, but also the records of the child in utero. Therefore, in addition to any legal rights that this daughter may have as next of kin, she may have some right of access to these records as records of her own health care.

A traditional consequentialist would ask whether the information would, on balance, be beneficial to the patient. It is apparent that the answer is not obvious. There is information at stake that is potentially important to her current health care. On the other hand, the physician and medical records administrator know what the patient probably does not. The information about the artificial insemination obviously could be potentially very upsetting to her and could affect her feelings about her deceased parents. Basing an assessment just on the consequences, what would you decide?

Now look at the case from the point of view of the rights of the patient. Assuming she has the right to information potentially meaningful in making medical decisions, does she have a right to the information even if it is, on balance, likely to harm her? The 1985 AMRA Code (IX, 2) stated that a medical record professional

> support and uphold the professional standards which will produce complete, accurate and timely information to meet the health and related needs of the patient and appropriate entities.[16]

The 1991 code of the American Health Information Management Association does not make such a commitment.

Does the physician's willingness to assure her that she was not exposed to diethylstilbestrol settle the matter or does she have a right to see the actual documents including the unexpected information?

ENDNOTES

1. Henry Sidgwick, *The Methods of Ethics* (New York: Dover, 1966; originally published, 1874).
2. Bernard Meyer, "Truth and the Physician," in *Ethical Issues in Medicine*, ed. E. Fuller Torrey (Boston: Little, Brown, 1968), pp. 159-177.
3. Immanuel Kant, "On the Supposed Right to Tell Lies from Benevolent Motives," trans. Thomas Kingsmill Abbott and reprinted in Kant's *Critique of Practical Reason and Other Works on the Theory of Ethics* (London: Longmans, 1909; originally published, 1797), pp. 361-365.
4. W. D. Ross, *The Right and the Good* (Oxford: Oxford University Press, 1939).
5. Donald Oken, "What to Tell Cancer Patients: A Study of Medical Attitudes," *Journal of the American Medical Association*, Vol. 175 (April 1, 1961), pp. 1120-1128.
6. Dennis H. Novack, Robin Plumer, Raymond L. Smith, Herbert Ochitill, Gary R. Morrow, and John M. Bennett, "Changes in Physicians' Attitudes Toward Telling the Cancer Patient," *Journal of the American Medical Association*, Vol. 241 (March 2, 1979), pp. 897-900.
7. The American Dietetic Association, *Code of Ethics for the Profession of Dietetics and Review Process for Alleged Violations* (Chicago: ADA, 1991).
8. American Occupational Therapy Association, *Occupational Therapy Code of Ethics*, 1994.
9. American Physical Therapy Association, *Guide for Professional Conduct* (Alexandria, VA: APTA, July 1991).
10. American Medical Association, *Principles of Medical Ethics of the American Medical Association*, published in *Journal of the American Medical Association*, Vol. 164 (1957), pp. 1119-1120. By contrast the AMA beginning with the principles published in 1981 commits the physician to deal honestly with patients. See American Medical Association, *Current Opinions of the Judicial Council of the American Medical Association* (Chicago: AMA, 1981).
11. American Academy of Physician Assistants, *Code of Ethics of the Physician Assistant Profession* (Alexandria, VA: AAPA, adopted 1983, amended 1985 House of Delegates).
12. American Society of Radiologic Technologists, *Code of Ethics*, revised Albuquerque, NM: July 1994).
13. The American Medical Records Association (AMRA), *Code of Ethics: Guide to the Interpretation of the Code of Ethics—1985 Revision*, published in *Journal of AMRA* (October 1987), pp. 57-58, provided an example. This code was changed in 1991 when the organization took on the name of the American Health Information Management Association.
14. American Society for Medical Technology, *Code of Ethics* (Washington, DC: ASMT, n.d.).
15. AMRA, AMRA *Code of Ethics—1985 Revision*.
16. Ibid.

CHAPTER 7

Fidelity

PROMISE-KEEPING AND CONFIDENTIALITY

The cases in the previous chapter presented a number of situations in which health care providers did not propose to overtly lie to patients, but nevertheless contemplated withholding the truth. We noted that the principle of veracity treated the intentional telling of false information as a moral infringement, but that it was less clear how to treat withholding of information. It seems clear that no one has a duty to tell all the truth to anyone who happens along. At the same time, certain people seem to have a duty not only to avoid lying, but also to tell certain things to others. In general, health providers who are in an ongoing relation with a patient or client have a duty to disclose to their patients or clients what they would reasonably want to know or find meaningful in making a decision related to care.

We might attribute such a duty to the principle of veracity (truthfulness, honesty, correctness, and accuracy), but it can also be associated with what we will call the principle of fidelity. When people exist in special relations with others, they take on special duties. Parents have duties to their children, spouses to each other, that they do not have with others. Likewise, when a health care provider enters a special relation with a patient or client, certain special obligations are created. As part of the contract or "covenant" that establishes the relation, commitments are made that generate new and special obligations. The duty to disclose potentially meaningful information is one such duty, but there are many others.

In general, when one party promises something to another, such a special relation is established. That promise can take the form of a routine promise to return something that has been borrowed, or it can take the form of establishing a relation between provider and client. Usually, promise-making is reciprocal. Each party offers something and agrees to be bound by mutual agreement. In health care, promises are made in scheduling appointments, in agreeing to fee schedules, and in keeping records. More fundamentally, promises are made when a client-provider relation is established that includes a provider's pledge of loyalty to the client—to abide by a code of ethics and to stay with the patient in time of need. Among the promises made is the promise to keep information confidential.

All promises are made with implicit or explicit limits. The commitment to establish a provider-client relation normally carries with it an implied limit that either party can break the relation under certain conditions: adequate notice, justifiable reason, and—in the case of the provider—arrangement for a colleague to assume responsibility.

The contract, covenant, commitment, or promise that establishes the relation between provider and client rests, in part, on the ethics of keeping promises. The principle underlying the idea that one has a duty—other things being equal—to keep a commitment once it is made is sometimes called the principle of fidelity. The cases in this chapter look at situations in which providers are faced with problems of what the moral limits are on keeping commitments once they are made. In particular, we will face cases in which the provider has made some sort of commitment and later discovers that, in the provider's estimate, the patient or someone else would be better off if the commitment were not kept. The general problem is, thus, one of the conflict between the principle of beneficence and the principle of fidelity.

The first cases involve general notions of fidelity to explicit and implicit promises. The second section of the chapter will deal with the more specific area of the promise of confidentiality and its limits. Finally, we will look at fidelity in terms of professional obligations and loyalty in terms of the problem of coping with an incompetent colleague.

THE ETHICS OF PROMISES: EXPLICIT AND IMPLICIT

We all learn very young that it is immoral to break a promise. Unfortunately, soon thereafter we also learn that there are cases when there are strong reasons why promises should not always be kept. Of course, there are promises that it is in one's self-interest to break. Normally, however, we do not confuse self-interest with reasons based on the welfare of others. These other-regarding reasons for breaking promises may pose a legitimate moral dilemma.

Sometimes, as in the first case in this section, the promise is explicit, and yet the one to whom the promise is made will be hurt only modestly if the promise is not kept and someone else will benefit enormously if it is violated. Does that count as an acceptable reason to break the promise in the following case?

CASE 38: Harmful Promises

Melinda Arons is a respiratory care practitioner in a small hospital. Sandy Smits is a 3-year-old suffering from smoke inhalation who is scheduled for several hours of ventilation support. Sandy was very afraid of the ventilator—her first time on such a machine. Sandy asks Ms. Arons to promise to stay with her throughout the entire treatment on the ventilator. Ms. Arons, without thinking, says, "of course."

Ninety minutes into the ventilator support therapy, there is a crisis elsewhere in the hospital. Ms. Arons is only one of two respiratory care practitioners on duty. The other patient has just arrived in the hospital having been involved in an automobile accident and having suffered a crushed chest. Should she leave Sandy to give treatment to the other patient when she has given her word to Sandy?

Look at Ms. Arons' problem first from the point of view of the likely benefits and harms of the alternatives. Certainly, Sandy might be upset if Ms. Arons leaves. On the other hand, she will probably recover from the unpleasantness and for the accident victim it could be a matter of life and death. From the utilitarian perspective, this would seem to be a case when more good could be done if the promise to Sandy is broken. Surely that would be the case if she were the only therapist on duty. Factoring in the other therapist may still lead to this conclusion.

Some utilitarians are what is called rule-utilitarians. They look at the moral rules governing human conduct and evaluate them on the basis of which general rules produce the best consequences. Then they apply the rule to the individual case without further assessment of the consequences in the individual case. Some do this out of concern that, especially in moments of crisis such as in a hospital setting, there will be too many errors in making complex calculations of benefits. Others do so just because they believe that morality is a matter of applying such rules to individual situations.

A rule-utilitarian would focus not on the specifics of this case and whether more good would be done if Ms. Arons broke her promise to Sandy, but rather on the general rule. In this case the rule might be something like, "When a promise is made, it ought to be kept." On the other hand, another possible rule could be, "Promises should be kept except when more good would be done by breaking the promise." The question is whether, in general, more good would come from following such a rule with the exception clause or from the rule that simply required that promises be kept whenever they are made. More good might come from the rule without the exceptions if we believed that those having to make split-second decisions in moments of crisis would make too many mistakes. More good might also come if those in the society realized that with the rule containing the exception clause, the entire practice of making promises would become tainted. People would always realize that the promise carried the exception clause, and therefore promise-making as a practice would be less useful. Further, as in the case just presented, could minors or incompetent patients understand either the rule or the exceptions?

Still others reject the whole idea of evaluating whether to keep a promise based on consequences (either assessing them in the specific situation or by looking at the consequences of alternative rules). Some, such as Immanuel Kant, hold that ethics is not a matter of consequences in either form. They believe that it is simply a moral wrong to break a promise—even if the consequences of breaking it would be better. For those who hold this view, we can say that part of the moral principle of fidelity is that it is simply right to keep promises and wrong to break them. Some who hold this view believe that fidelity is only a *prima facie* principle—that is, it indicates a relevant moral dimension of the situation—but that it could be overridden by other moral principles. In this case, the overriding principle would probably have to be beneficence.

Under what conditions, if any, can Ms. Arons' promise to Sandy be broken? For instance, in the case of an adult we might be able to ask the patient for permission to leave for a while. If the one making the promise is released by the one to whom the promise is made, then surely there is no longer a moral duty to keep the promise. But Sandy is only 3 years old. Can she understand and release Ms. Arons? Is there any other moral basis on which to justify leaving Sandy?

Sometimes the promise made is less explicit than in the previous case. Commitments can be implied or based on what is customary in relationships. In establishing a relationship with a patient or client in health care, many assumptions are made that may have the effect of making commitments between the parties. Patients who have potentially interesting histories are potential sources of curiosity for many who have no professional need to know the details. The following case poses the question of the moral commitment made to a patient who could provide some interesting gossip for a respiratory care practitioner.

CASE 39: Gossip and Fidelity to the Patient

Mary Still is a respiratory care practitioner in a small hospital. She has just learned that the daughter of the president of the local university has been assigned for treatment. Shortly after Ms. Still completes the first treatment of her new patient, inquiries come forth from her colleagues. They want to know what Mary's new patient is like.

When Mary goes home, she receives a phone call from her mother who asks her about the president's daughter and if the president has come in. It seems that the gossip about the city was that the president's daughter had been raped. Everyone who calls wants to know about this.

What is at stake here is exactly what commitment Ms. Still makes when she enters into a relation with her patient. The question could be approached by asking what the content of the various professional codes is. In the case of respiratory care, for example, the American Association for Respiratory Care *Code of Ethics* requires that the respiratory care practitioner "shall hold in strict confidence all privileged information concerning the patient and refer all inquiries to the physician in charge of the patient's medical care."[1] Do such restrictions and requirements apply to confidence keeping outside the realm of the health care institution?

While there is general agreement that there is a duty of health professionals to protect confidentiality, we shall see in the next section that the exact basis and limits on that duty are unclear. Ms. Still might ask why she is morally bound not to disclose details about the case simply because her professional association says so. The question is even more pressing when we realize that many other allied health professional codes have somewhat different positions on confidentiality. For example, the 1988 version of the *Occupational Therapy Code of Ethics* required confidence keeping or fidelity "unless sharing such information could be deemed necessary to protect the well-being of a third party."[2] The American Society of Radiologic Technology *Code of Ethics*—like that of the Respiratory Care Association—requires that all information regarding patients be held in strict confidence.[3] Even more important, people who are not members of these associations may also have opinions on the ethics of disclosing personal information of the sort in this case.

The principle of fidelity probably provides the best underpinning of the duty not to disclose information learned in personal relations. The general idea is that by establishing a relation with another, you make certain commitments—implied promises—including the promise not to disclose to outsiders such personal knowledge you gain as a result of the faith the other puts in you. This applies not only to professional relations such as those of the respiratory care practitioner, but to friendships as well.

In the case of the health care provider, the promise is made more explicit. At least if Ms. Still is a member of her professional association, she presumably subscribes to its code of ethics. That does not provide the ultimate reason why it is wrong for her to discuss the details of her patient's case, but it does mean that if she does not feel bound by the commitment, she has a duty to let the patient know. Assuming that she has not told the patient she has rejected the professional code, she has, in effect, promised to the patient that she will not discuss the details of her personal history, at least without good reason. The cases in the next section look at what, if anything, would count as a good reason for disclosing confidential information.

THE LIMITS ON THE PROMISE OF CONFIDENTIALITY

As already alluded to, an allied health professional code may provide exceptions to confidentiality. As in Case 38, in which a respiratory care practitioner promised to stay with a young patient on a ventilator only to discover that she was desperately needed by another patient in more dire straits, sometimes people discover reasons why they might consider wanting to break the promise of confidentiality. Two general reasons arise: breaking confidence to benefit the patient and breaking it to benefit others.

1. Breaking Confidence to Benefit the Patient

In Case 39, whatever reason the respiratory care practitioner had to disclose information about her patient, it clearly was not for the patient's benefit. Sometimes, however, a health care provider comes to believe that the patient very much needs to have someone else know some important, but perhaps embarrassing or controversial, fact. If the patient agrees to the disclosure there is no problem, but what happens, as in the following two cases, when the patient refuses to agree?

CASE 40: Disclosing a Psychiatric Patient's Medications to His Family

The following incident is described by James Austin, second-year occupational therapy student.

"Wallace Hanson is a 25-year-old male who lives with his parents in Johnson County, Illinois. Mr. Hanson was brought to the locked psychiatric unit of a private hospital after a temporary detention order was sought by his parents. His parents claimed that he was saying things that didn't make sense, threatening violence against them, and throwing things in the house. A hearing was scheduled to determine whether he should be held for treatment. His parents came to the hospital for the hearing. While they were waiting, they asked to speak to the occupational therapist. The reasons for meeting with a family prior to a commitment hearing are many. To help them understand the process involved and what treatment awaits their family member if he is or is not committed, to clear up any questions about insurance coverage, and to begin to work on the issue of whether a living situation will need to be arranged prior to discharge are but a few of the possible reasons for such a meeting. In this case, all these things were addressed. He would be needing a place to live because the family was not willing to take him back into their home. Insurance coverage was intact, so the patient would be able to stay in the private hospital if committed. His mother also used this meeting to ask about medication. She had knowledge of some medications working better than others and of some medications causing negative reactions in her son's case. We spoke of how he had been doing since coming to the hospital, and I gave her information regarding which medications he was taking in the hospital.

"The ethical issue involved here is: When, in a hospital setting, is it permissible to speak on the client's behalf to significant others without the client's permission? In this case, I had not obtained his permission to do this mainly for reasons of expediency. In other cases, a patient may be disorganized in his thinking, angry, or even violent toward the person that had him brought to the hospital against his will and will not give the occupational therapist permission to make such contacts, if asked. If the person is in a state of paranoid thinking, the thought of the occupational therapist calling his significant others to ask about the patient may be a very threatening notion. Such contacts are often necessary in order to get a clear picture of the patient's normal and abnormal functioning, so as to be able to provide quality care.

"It is my position that if, in the clinical judgment of the occupational therapist, the patient is incompetent to give his permission, or to withhold it for a rational reason, the occupational therapist should make this decision himself or herself, in the best interest of the patient. If, in the judgment of the therapist, asking permission would be countertherapeutic, as in the case of the person with paranoid thinking, such a request should be forgone, the reasons should be documented, and the occupational therapist should proceed.

"After having given Mr. Hanson's mother the name and dosages of his medications, I was informed by a registered nurse in the unit that the mother had also asked her the same information and that she had refused to give her that information because she did not have the patient's permission. She also informed me that I may have put myself in legal jeopardy if the patient ever decided to make a case out of it."

This student might, at first, assume that Mr. Hanson's mother is his guardian or that, at least, she is authorized to make medical decisions on his behalf. If the patient has been determined to be incompetent, the guardian of the patient, if one has been designated, must have access to information in order to consent or refuse consent to treatment on the patient's behalf.

But there is nothing in this case that establishes either that the patient has been declared incompetent or that his mother has been designated his guardian. Notice that the occupational therapy student took the position that "If, in the clinical judgment of the occupational therapist, the patient is incompetent to give his permission or to withhold it for a rational reason, the occupational therapist should make this decision him or herself." Mr. Austin's assumption is that not only can he decide the patient is incompetent, but that he can determine whether the patient should be informed that a decision is being made to disclose information of a confidential nature. Competency, however, is a legal determination. In fact it is the hearing that is about to be held that will likely, among other things, determine Mr. Hanson's competence. The temporary commitment order, in most jurisdictions, does not involve a full competency determination. Even if Mr. Hanson were determined to be incompetent, it is not clear that his mother would be appointed his guardian. She and her husband may be devoted and concerned about their son's well-being, but they have sought to have him committed and have decided that he cannot return to their house. It appears that they do not necessarily have a claim to the information on the grounds that they are his guardians.

But Mr. Austin could still be convinced that it is in Mr. Hanson's interest for his parents to know what medication he is on. They may know about idiosyncratic side effects that have bothered him in the past or of medication that has been particularly effective. How realistic is it for the occupational therapy student to believe that Mr. Hanson's interest would be served if his parents knew which medication he was taking?

Assuming that the occupational therapy student's belief is plausible, there are additional problems. First, note that this is a student, not a graduate occupational therapist. What steps should a student take who believes his or her patient should be treated in a certain way? Should the treatment intervention (in this case, the disclosure of information) be approved by the supervising practitioner?

Finally, examine the substantive issue itself. Assuming that the supervising occupational therapist concurred that it would be in the patient's interest to have the information transmitted to Mr. Hanson's parents even though they were not legally his guardians, would it be ethical to tell them the information and to fail to reveal this to Mr. Hanson? Does this situation fit the exception clause stated in the professional code for occupational therapists when it says that, "The individual shall protect the confidential nature of information gained from educational, practice, and investigational activities unless sharing such information could be deemed necessary to protect the well-being of a third party"?[4] That would seem to justify breaking a confidence to protect the parents, but not to protect the patient himself. Suppose Mr. Hanson's parents had asked the physician assistant on the health care team. Its code authorizes breaking confidence not only to protect third parties, but to protect the patient as well.[5] Can it simultaneously be wrong for some members of the team to disclose the medications and right for other members?

Many of the traditional ethical codes in the health professions take their lead from the Hippocratic Oath. They provide an exception to the confidentiality rule in cases in which the health care provider believes that the patient would benefit from disclosure. As in the occupational therapy student's case, they even accept such disclosure without informing the patient if the health care provider believes it would be contraindicated or, as the student says, "countertherapeutic."

The physician assistant code, as we have seen, says that confidentiality shall be upheld unless "such information becomes necessary to protect the welfare of the patient ..."[6] Other codes, such as those of the medical technologists,[7] commit their members to an absolute, exceptionless pledge of confidentiality, not even permitting breaking confidence when there appears to be a serious threat of harm to others.

The physician assistants' code is traditionally paternalistic. It would let the consequences alone determine whether information should be disclosed. The other codes appear to be abandoning consequentialist reasoning. They seem to hold that breaking a confidence is always wrong no matter what the consequences for the patient. Which reasoning was the occupational therapy student using? Should the health care provider's position on confidentiality depend on which professional group he or she happens to belong to? What promise, implied or explicit, is made to a patient in this situation about the confidentiality of medical information?

CASE 41: Parental Access to an Infant's Medical Record

A man arrived at the hospital Medical Records Department requesting to review the record of his newborn son, delivered to his wife three weeks earlier. The man signed the authorization form prepared by the release-of-information secretary, who asked him to wait while she went to locate the record. Upon obtaining the newborn's record, the release-of-information secretary reviewed the record privately in accordance with hospital policy to make sure the record was complete and not related to any current litigation involving the hospital. Hospital policy specifies that incomplete records are not available for release until completion and records involved in litigation involving the hospital require notification of risk management prior to release. Release-of-information policies also provide for access to or authorization for release by parents to patient record information of their minor children.

The hospital's patient record system routinely maintains separate records for mother and newborn; however, a copy of the birth certificate is retained in both records. Upon review of the baby's record, the release-of-information secretary notes that the birth certificate, completed in accordance with information supplied by the mother, indicates that the baby's father is a man whose name is not the same as that on the authorization just signed. The release-of-information secretary returns to the requestor without the record, asking for verification of his identity and whether he uses any other name. These requests are presented as routine. The man denies any aliases and can provide suitable identification, but he also becomes agitated and insists that he wants to review his son's record immediately.

This case involves issues both of the right of access to information (issues discussed in Chapter 6) and the right of confidentiality. In contrast with the previous case, the man who presents himself as the father and who presumably believes he is the father is legally authorized to act as the surrogate for his son—assuming it is his son. Thus, the problem of the parent's right of access is not raised upon the initial request for the record. But it is less clear what is required legally or ethically if the mother has led him to believe that he is the father and that he, in fact, will play the role of the father, but in reality he is not. Has the mother, by letting him believe he is the father, actually authorized him to have the rights to the records that he would have if he were the father?

The release-of-information secretary is in a difficult position. She is prepared to give the record to the father, but she has a duty to protect the confidentiality of the mother's record. She also has a duty to protect the infant's record from those who have no right to see it. But merely telling the man who is the purported father that he may not have a right to see the record will break the confidentiality, in effect disclosing what the mother would most want kept secret.

What would constitute the interests of the infant, the mother, and her husband in this case? Does the real father, assuming it is not the husband, have a right to insist that the record be kept confidential? Should the records secretary approach the problem focusing on the welfare of her patient and, if so, who is (or are) her patient? Is this a case that should be settled by trying to promote the welfare of the patient, by trying to maximize the net of benefit minus harm taking into account all parties, or by appealing to certain rights grounded in promises made or duties of fidelity?

This type of case is a problem from a medical record practitioner perspective. Lying about medical record content under most circumstances is pointless because the record can usually be obtained legally by an authorized individual to verify the information; tampering with or alteration of information in a patient record is regarded as a cardinal sin for medical records administrators. The American Health Information Management Association *Code of Ethics* states that a member professional should ensure release of information only if it is in accordance with current laws and regulations and institutional policies."[8] But the release-of-information secretary may want to know what is ethical, not merely what is in accord with current laws and regulations and institutional policies.

2. Breaking Confidence to Benefit Others

While breaking confidence paternalistically to benefit the patient is one of the traditional justifications for disclosure, serving the welfare of other parties is the second. According to a rigid application of the traditional Hippocratic ethic, all actions of the health care provider should be solely for the welfare of the patient. Of course, this means that any action for the purpose of serving other individuals or the society as a whole would be unethical. This would make unethical not only public health interventions, research medicine, and cost containment, but would also make it unethical to disclose confidential information for the benefit of another. In the array of codes of ethics of allied health professionals we have quite a variation of statements concerning the matter of breaking confidence in order to benefit others. For instance, the occupational therapist code simply pledged confidentiality without exception.[9] The physician assistant code permits breaking of confidence to benefit third parties as well as the patient.[10] The radiologic technologist code permits breaking confidence to benefit third parties.[11]

The following case poses the question of whether the promise made by the health care provider should be to keep medical information confidential no matter what or should contain an exception when there are risks to others that can only be prevented by breaking a confidence.

CASE 42: Confidentiality When Others May Be Harmed

Memorial Hospital's laboratory has just received a contract to serve as one of the testing sites for the State Department of Health for the human immunodeficiency virus (HIV). The state has mandated an anonymous program with the use of code numbers that the individuals to be tested determine for themselves. Results of the tests are provided to individuals upon presentation of their half of the coded request form.

The technologist responsible for the testing unit has determined that a blind quality control (QC) program is important in addition to the usual QC activities. Her blind testing program consists of the submission of samples to the lab of bloods from healthy persons (usually other laboratory staff). These results are monitored closely to ascertain the consistency of results. Only the supervisor knows which samples are quality control samples, and she is the only person who sees all the results.

In addition to general adherence to the ethical principle of confidentiality, the laboratory has sworn in their state contract to preserve the confidentiality of all acquired immune deficiency syndrome (AIDS) testing information. Positive test results are accompanied by an information package and a request that the individual seek the assistance of a physician; however, no attempt is made to identify the person. The state receives reports for epidemiologic purposes, which contain numerical data on numbers of tests, positive and negative results, age, and gender.

When one of the quality control samples unexpectedly yielded positive results, the supervisor was presented with a real dilemma. She was aware of the identity of the individual and knew her to be a married woman with young children. She was not in any of the high-risk groups and was, therefore, certain that she was negative for the HIV antibody.

Believing that the results were an error and that there may be a quality control problem, the supervisor obtained another blood sample and submitted it for testing. Again the results were positive.

What should the supervisor do? Having sworn to maintain the confidentiality of all persons being tested, how could she violate the oath by discussing these results even with the person herself? If the employee refuses to disclose the results to her husband, then what would the lab supervisor's obligation be? Sharing the information would violate the rules of confidentiality. However, not sharing the information increased the risk to her husband and diminished her likelihood of effective treatment because of treatment delay. Is confidentiality more important than offering help to others who need the confidential medical information?

The case reveals the problem that can be created if the wrong promise is made. If the state contract would forbid disclosure to anyone, even the one being tested, then surely that is not a wise commitment to which to agree. In fact, because the individuals being tested as patients rather than as quality controls get their results, the implication is that the state contract does not envision withholding the results even from the one who supplied the sample.

This case, however, suggests there was something wrong with the collection of the blind samples. If they were submitted using the same procedures, the laboratory staff should know the samples only by their code numbers; they should not know who the source was. Apparently for the controls, the identity of the source was kept from the technologist responsible for doing the analysis, but it was apparently not kept from the supervisor conducting the test. Were the laboratory staff and others supplying the control samples misled here?

A more substantial problem arises if the employee or anyone else who tests positive for HIV admits that he or she is exposing others to risks and refuses to disclose that fact to contacts. In this case, if the employee refuses to disclose the risk, an argument can be made that the health care provider, in this case the laboratory technologist, has a moral duty to protect the ones at risk by warning them.

In one famous California court case, a psychologist who had been told by a patient that he planned to murder a former girlfriend was found to have a duty to warn notwithstanding the traditional professional ethical duty of confidentiality.[12] It was important in that decision that the psychologist was himself convinced that his patient was going to carry out the threat and that the risk was a substantial one.

In the discussion of Case 40 it can be seen that some codes of allied health professions have reacted to the excessive paternalism of the Hippocratic tradition by making a flat, exceptionless commitment to confidentiality. We saw that response in the medical technologists' *Code of Ethics* and the occupational therapists' *Code of Ethics*. They, however, are now committed to a blank-check promise of nondisclosure no matter what the gravity of the risk to others.

By contrast the American Physical Therapy Association permits disclosure "to appropriate authorities when it is necessary to protect the welfare of an individual or the community."[13] This, taken at face value, would open the door quite wide for disclosures. The Physical Therapy Association, however, limits disclosure by adding, "Such disclosure shall be in accordance with applicable law." In effect this says that whatever is legal is ethical and only whatever is legal. Since the state of the law is ambiguous and, at least in the case of serious threats of injury, disclosure may actually be required by law, it is not clear that this qualifier will constrain the broad exception based on the welfare of the community for physical therapists choosing to conform to their association's code.

Many professional groups and many laypeople reflecting on this problem have concluded that, while trivial concerns about the welfare of the community surely should not justify breaking confidence, some risks to others are so great that they must be reported. In fact the law requires some health professionals to report such risks as diagnosis of venereal disease, gunshot wounds, and child abuse. The American Medical Association has changed its code of ethics to permit (or perhaps require) disclosure when "a patient threatens to inflict serious bodily harm to another person and there is a reasonable probability that the patient may carry out the threat."[14]

If the supervising technologist is going to resolve this problem, she will need to be clear on exactly what she has promised—either in the process of being licensed or in the process of negotiating the contract and recruiting the employee to provide the blood sample. What would be an appropriate promise to make regarding the discovery that an employee tests positive? Would the risk to her husband if she refuses to tell him be so severe that the technologist should avoid promising to keep the diagnosis secret if the employee remains silent or is confidentiality among co-workers so important that even this kind of risk to the husband should not justify telling him?

INCOMPETENT AND DISHONEST COLLEAGUES

The principle of fidelity has thus far been applied to the areas of the making and breaking of promises and, in particular, the keeping of confidences. Those who recognize an independent principle of fidelity believe that there is something intrinsically immoral about breaking a promise, including the promise to keep medical information confidential.

There are other implications of the principle of fidelity. One of the most significant regards loyalty to colleagues, especially when it conflicts with loyalty to the profession and to the patient. Many of the professional codes require reporting of incompetent or dishonest practices. This seems consistent with serving the welfare of patients as well as showing loyalty to the profession of which one is a member. However, we are also expected in life to be loyal to our friends and colleagues. If a colleague appears to be incompetent or dishonest, as in the following case, the health care worker is often put in an impossible situation.

CASE 43: Reporting a Colleague Who Cheats a Patient

Ann Taylor is a respiratory care practitioner in a large hospital. In the respiratory care service office, she observes her colleague, Will Marshall, recording treatments in the chart of Mrs. Mildred Brown who is a roommate of one of Ms. Taylor's patients, Mrs. Delores Harris.

About a half hour later, Ms. Taylor visits Mrs. Harris' room to check her oxygen. Mrs. Brown, who is awake, asks Ms. Taylor, "When is Mr. Marshall going to come for my treatment? The day is almost gone."

Ms. Taylor and Mr. Marshall have always been very close. This is not the first time that there have been allegations that Mr. Marshall has not given all the treatments that he should. Ms. Taylor is in a dilemma. What should she do? If she goes to the supervisor, Mr. Marshall could lose his job.*

Ann Taylor appears to have caught her colleague, Will Marshall, red-handed. He has not only cheated his patient and her insurer, but he has also risked her health. Are there any other explanations for what she has seen? Could he have forgotten to provide the therapy?

**This case was supplied by Professor Leslie Elder.*

In either case, Ms. Taylor is facing a problem. Mr. Marshall is either dishonest or incompetent. If the pattern is persisting, as apparently it is, the mere fact that the omissions were an accident would not relieve Ms. Taylor of her responsibility to protect her patient. What difference does it make morally if Mr. Marshall forgot or intentionally omitted the treatments?

What does the principle of fidelity or loyalty require here? Ms. Taylor may think of herself as having made commitments to the patient, the profession, and her colleague. Is it to the patient, the profession, or one's colleagues that one is accountable? Consider the following options. Which should she choose?

1. Report Mr. Marshall to her supervisor even though he will risk losing his job.
2. Speak directly to him to see if his performance changes.
3. Report to the patient's physician that the care is apparently not being provided.
4. Inform the patient of the omission of the therapy and the erroneous recording in the chart.
5. Discuss the problem with other members of the health care team.
6. Remain silent and stay out of trouble.

ENDNOTES

1. American Association for Respiratory Care, *Code of Ethics* (Dallas, TX: AARC, n.d.).
2. American Occupational Therapy Association (AOTA), *Occupational Therapy Code of Ethics*, 1988.
3. American Society of Radiologic Technology (ASRT), *Code of Ethics* (Albuquerque, NM: ASRT, 1994).
4. AOTA, *Occupational Therapy Code of Ethics.*
5. American Academy of Physician Assistants (AAPA), *Code of Ethics of the Physician Assistant Profession* (Alexandria, VA: AAPA, adopted 1983, amended 1985 House of Delegates).
6. Ibid.
7. ASRT, *Code of Ethics.*
8. American Health Information Management Association, *AHIMA Code of Ethics*, 1991.
9. AOTA, *Occupational Therapy Code of Ethics*, 1994.
10. AAPA, *Code of Ethics of the Physician Assistant Profession.*
11. ASRT, *Code of Ethics*, 1994.

12. *Tarasoff* v. *Regents of University of California*, 17C.3d 425, 131 Cal. Rptr. 14, 551 P.2d 334, in Thomas A. Shannon and Jo Ann Manfra, eds., *Law and Bioethics: Texts with Commentary on Major U.S. Court Decisions* (New York: Paulist Press, 1982), pp. 293-319.
13. American Physical Therapy Association, *Guide for Professional Conduct* (Alexandria, VA: APTA, July 1994).
14. American Medical Association, Judicial Council, *Current Opinions of the Council on Ethical and Judicial Affairs of the American Medical Association: Including the Principles of Medical Ethics and Rules of the Council on Ethical and Judicial Affairs* (Chicago: AMA, 1989), p. 21.

CHAPTER 8

Avoidance of Killing

The principles examined in the preceding chapters—beneficence, nonmaleficence, justice, autonomy, veracity, and fidelity—cover most of the moral considerations that arise in one-on-one personal moral decisions involving allied health professionals. But before turning to some special topical areas in Part III, we should look at one additional moral consideration at the level of the individual. Many moral controversies in health care hinge on claims that are variously based on the notion that human life is sacred or that killing of a human is morally wrong. In this chapter, we shall look at cases involving allied health professionals who are put in positions in which they need to know exactly what is implied by these notions.

For all of us, killing of another is usually wrong if for no other reason than that normally people want to live. Killing does people harm in a dramatic way. The principle of nonmaleficence (not harming) counts strongly against killing in most cases. But there are special cases when it is not as obvious that killing would be perceived as a harm by the individual. Some patients are suicidal. Others are so racked with the pain of a chronic, perhaps terminal, illness that the patient would plead to be killed or to be aided in dying.

Our traditional religious and secular values have dictated that even in these cases it is wrong to kill. But why? If the killing relieves severe suffering, can it not count as a good and noble thing to help those who are suffering end it?

Some people hold that in ethics, the consequences are the only relevant factor. Utilitarians, for example, hold this view. So do those who subscribe to the Hippocratic principle, which requires the health professional to always act only so as to benefit the patient. Although many health providers do not realize it, the Hippocratic principle by itself could permit or even require the health provider to cooperate in killing a patient when it would, on balance, do more good than harm.

But the Hippocratic Oath also contains a specific provision that is usually interpreted as prohibiting active killing. Technically, it proscribes "giving a deadly drug, even if asked." But usually in modern readings, that is taken to generally prohibit any physician participation in killing. Insofar as the oath can be extended to all health professionals, it would prohibit allied health professionals from participating as well. Since most allied health professionals are not normally in positions where they would seriously contemplate killing patients on their own, the codes of the allied health professions generally do not mention a prohibition on killing, but one can assume that such actions would be opposed by the traditional allied health professional organizations. In fact, as we shall see in the cases in this chapter, allied health professionals do actually encounter situations where they are at least asked to cooperate in forgoing life-sustaining treatment and sometimes they are actually placed in positions where they could consider whether to kill actively.

The interesting problem is why such a prohibition on killing exists if the goal of the provider is always to benefit the patient. One possibility, of course, would be that the authors of the oath considered it always a net harm to the patient to end the patient's life. Many people, however, are willing to concede that at least in rare cases the patient may be worse off if he or she continues to live. If that is true, then there are two other possible justifications for proscribing merciful killings.

First, as we have seen in previous chapters, some people who base moral judgments on consequences do not believe it is right to directly calculate the consequences in each individual case. Instead, they consider possible alternative moral rules or policies. They assess the net consequences of the alternative rules or policies and choose the rule or policy that they believe will do more good than any alternative. These people are usually called *rule-utilitarians*.[1]

They may do this for a number of reasons. First, some are worried about the risk of error if individuals were permitted to make the calculations on the spot for each case. Especially in highly emotionally charged situations where rapid decisions have to be made and especially when those doing the calculating may not know the individuals affected very well, the danger of miscalculation may be great. They believe that in the long run more good may be done (and more harm prevented) if we simply apply the rule chosen because on balance it will produce more good than any alternative.

Second, some people, not necessarily persuaded that the risk of error is this great, may still hold that it is just the nature of morality that practices are established by evaluating alternative rules or policies and choosing the set that produces the greatest net good.[2] For either of these reasons, some consequentialists, those who are rule-consequentialists, may favor a rule that prohibits the participation of health professionals in killing.

There is a second reason why the Hippocratic Oath may prohibit active killings for mercy. As we have seen in previous chapters, there may be moral principles other than beneficence and nonmaleficence that determine whether an act is right or wrong. We have already seen that some people hold that autonomy, veracity, and fidelity to promises help determine the rightness of actions regardless of the consequences. Is it possible that killing is just inherently wrong—even if the one who is killed is better off than if he or she had lived? If so, avoidance of killing could be an independent principle that helps shape the rightness and wrongness of human conduct. We might refer to it simply as the principle of avoidance of killing. It is not clear whether the writer of the Hippocratic Oath believed this. If he did, then he is not a pure consequentialist.

Whether the Hippocratic author believes that killing people is inherently wrong, clearly other moral traditions are committed to this view. Judaism considers life to be sacred, a gift from God. Killing a human, at least an innocent human, is always wrong. Likewise, Catholicism considers killing an intrinsic wrong. Other moral traditions, both religious and secular, do as well.[3] If killing is always a wrong-making characteristic, then avoidance of killing can be thought of as another moral principle that must hold beneficence and nonmaleficence in check.[4] The cases in this chapter help to clarify how allied health professionals should evaluate possible attempts to relieve patients of their misery by putting them to death. In later sections of the chapter, participation in active merciful killing will be compared with decisions to forgo treatment (to withhold or withdraw treatment).

ACTIVE KILLING VERSUS LETTING DIE

Both religious and secular traditions in the West hold that it is always morally wrong to actively kill a human being even if the killing is done for a merciful motive. For example, some terminally ill patients appear to be in pain. If they are inevitably dying rapidly and could be spared the misery of the dying if someone simply actively intervened with an injection of a drug to hasten the death, some argue that such intervention would be the humane and moral thing to do. But others claim that there is something intrinsically wrong with killing—that life is sacred and to be preserved or that at least it should not be ended directly by human hand. The following two cases raise the question of whether there is any significant moral difference between actively killing someone who is dying and simply stepping aside and letting nature take its course.

CASE 44: Actively Ending the Agony

This is the fifth hospitalization of Cindy, a frail 22-month-old who presents with severe shortness of breath and congestion. The patient is extremely thin, her skin is covered with reddish lesions, and she appears very uncomfortable and exhausted. Only low whispers and moans are audible from the child. Her mother is in tears and has requested a private meeting with Donald Harvester, the PA.

During the meeting she explains, "My daughter does not deserve this pain and suffering. She has been sick most of her life and has not been able to run and play like other children. Her father died when she was 2 months old, and I didn't know he had AIDS until afterwards." (With loud crying, the mother continues.) "Now I've got it, and my daughter's got it. You've got to help me. I can't stand to see Cindy suffer like this."

The PA explains that "It's just a matter of time, we're doing all we can to help your daughter." The mother then says, "Please stop this, I know you can." Reaching into her purse, she pulls out a vial of street narcotics. She then pleads with the PA to administer the drugs through the intravenous catheter. "No one has to know about this. It's not right for my baby to suffer. Please, you've got to help."

The PA reflects on his role and is torn between the desire to alleviate suffering on one hand and to "do no harm" on the other. As a father of young children he feels emotional about this case.

Donald Harvester, the PA in this case, realizes that he has in his power the capacity to permanently end this baby's suffering and to put this mother's mind at ease. He should also realize that what is being proposed is illegal. The law does not settle the underlying ethical issues raised by the case, however. Some things that are ethical turn out to be illegal, while others that are legal may still be unethical.

Mr. Harvester may be contemplating whether this is the moment for an act of civil disobedience, purposely violating the civil law in order to conform to a higher law. Or he may be contemplating the public policy question currently being debated in state legislatures and national parliaments: Should the current law be changed to legalize merciful killing and, if so, under what circumstances?

One approach to these issues focuses on the consequences. It is striking that Mr. Harvester reaches for one of the slogans of traditional professional medical ethics, the maxim "Do no harm." It is precisely this question—whether killing a baby in Cindy's condition really is "doing harm"—that is currently controversial. Defenders of the morality of mercy killing argue that, far from hurting her, an active administration of the drug would spare her further harm. On the other hand, some people claim that life is precious—an intrinsically good thing—so that ending it is always doing a harm even if it also eliminates future suffering in the process. If one is a pure consequentialist, then the critical question is whether killing does more good or harm.

Defenders of active killing claim that killing does no harm in such cases and may actually prevent future harm. They argue that, if the active intervention shortens the period of suffering, it may actually be morally preferred over simply stepping back and letting the patient die.

Critics of such practices also raise arguments based in consequences. They claim that the consequences of a policy authorizing active killing may be different from those of a policy that accepts the forgoing of life-sustaining treatment. Some of these critics are what in the introduction we called *rule-utilitarians*. They believe that morality is based on certain practices or rules. They assess the consequences of the general rules rather than those of specific choices in individual cases. They believe that even if Mr. Harvester and Cindy's mother can correctly determine the consequences in this case, the risk of abuse of a policy endorsing active killing is too great. They worry that eventually those who are unwanted, unloved, or unattached to others will be done away with through misguided or uncaring decisions to kill in a purportedly merciful way. Particularly in cases such as Cindy, who at 22 months surely cannot speak for herself on the matter, they believe that the risks of others being permitted to determine that people would be better off dead are simply too great.

Deontologists believe there is more to morality than simply calculating consequences. They believe that certain characteristics of actions—such as lying or breaking promises—make actions wrong even if they would produce better consequences than alternative actions. Some people approach the question of mercy killing from the same perspective. They believe that calculating the consequences of killing for mercy will not necessarily settle the matter.

There are those who believe that killing another human is simply wrong, regardless of whether it relieves suffering. This principle is sometimes expressed, especially by the religious, as the principle of the sacredness of life. Holders of this view, however, must confront the issue of whether it is equally wrong to forgo life-sustaining treatment when doing so will have the result of a quicker death. Some people, for instance some

Jews, hold that life is sacred in its every moment, so that forgoing life-sustaining treatment is just as wrong as actively killing.

Others, such as many Catholics, affirm that forgoing life-sustaining treatment is morally acceptable if the intention is not to kill the patient, but only to remove treatment that no longer fits the patient's condition. They sometimes say that the withdrawal of the treatment does not kill that patient, the underlying disease does (even though, if they are honest, they admit that the patient would have died differently and not as quickly had the life-sustaining intervention been continued).

Those who see active killing as intrinsically wrong could be said to include an additional principle in their list of right-making characteristics along with veracity, autonomy, and fidelity. They could be said to also include the principle of avoidance of killing. This could include a prohibition on both active killing and forgoing treatment or, as is common in the United States and much ethical thinking, extend only to prohibiting active killing. Mr. Harvester must consider whether the consequences of killing this child are really going to be better, as the mother contends; whether he needs to be concerned about the general rule or only the individual case; and, finally, whether there is a principle that prohibits active killing even if it will be better for this patient.

The ethics of active killing in the health professions is not limited to cases such as the previous one where the killing is contemplated to show mercy to the patient. Although health providers are not normally asked to cooperate in killing for the good of the society, there are such cases. The issue arises in the military, and also, as in the following case, in medical means of capital punishment.

CASE 45: The Health Provider as Executioner

PA Janet Foxx is a new graduate and employee in the medical services division for the Department of Corrections. She has worked hard to earn a good reputation, and all work reports thus far have been superior. Being pleased with her performance, her supervising physician has offered an increase in salary and an upgrade in her professional duties.

One of her new duties will include working on death row. Now that the death penalty has been reinstated, executions by lethal injection will begin next week. Since physician assistant duties include administration of medication by injection, PA Foxx has been detailed to administer the lethal injections to inmates.

PA Foxx enjoys her job and wants to continue receiving a good report. She has no reservations about her technical ability to give the injections, but is unsure about taking a person's life. She feels somewhat confused about her role and questions if the injection could be given by the correctional officer. The correctional staff states that injections are clearly the role of the medical staff. (Note: The American Academy of Physician Assistants recently developed a position paper against lethal injections.)

This case raises all the issues about the ethics of killing that emerged in Case 44, but raises some additional questions as well. Whatever one thinks about mercy killing, it is consistent with the traditional health care ethic of striving to do what one believes will benefit the patient. Ms. Foxx's situation, however, is quite different in this regard. She is contemplating a killing that is not for the prisoner's benefit but, presumably, for the benefit of the society. It is either to punish for previous offense or to deter future offenses.

A traditional social utilitarian will not be troubled by this difference. Such a utilitarian calculates whether an action is morally acceptable based on the total consequences for all affected parties. The effect on the patient is presumably negative, but that must be combined with the effect on others according to a social utilitarian. If the benefits to others offset the harm to the individual, then the killing would be justified. A utilitarian possibly would oppose capital punishment solely to punish, but would support it if he or she believed it would produce the good result of deterring future antisocial actions.

There is another difference between the two cases that could be relevant even to deontologists who believe that there is a principle of avoidance of killing that simply prohibits killing (even when the net effects are an increase in welfare for the community). Traditionally, those who have held that it is wrong to kill have sometimes limited this principle to the killing of the innocent. While patients who might be killed for mercy are innocent, presumably a prisoner who has been sentenced to a capital punishment is not. If the prohibition on killing applies only to the innocent, that would justify killing in war, in self-defense, and, arguably, as a punishment.

Critics of capital punishment sometimes argue consequentially that there is no evidence that it works. Deontologists who are focusing on other moral dimensions may, however, be more concerned about "just deserts" than about the consequences. Still, some deontologists hold that the principle of avoidance of killing applies to all parties, at least *prima facie*. They might acknowledge that when this principle conflicts with others, the others may be overriding, but they would hold that it is wrong to kill, and sometimes that extends even to killing of those who are not innocent.

This raises one final question. Even if killing for mercy or killing for societal purposes turns out to be ethical, it does not follow that health professionals should be the ones who do the killing. There are some reasons why they would be good at it; they certainly have the relevant knowledge and skills. But others argue that regardless of their abilities, health care providers are in roles that are incompatible with killing. Their duty is to heal—to cure, relieve suffering, and promote health—but not to use their skills to purposely end life. This has been interpreted as prohibiting both killing for mercy and killing for corporal punishment as well as cooperation in the military enterprise. Should Ms. Foxx view the new assignment as outside the scope of what moral physician assistants can provide—even if it costs her the promotion?

WITHHOLDING VERSUS WITHDRAWING TREATMENT

While the distinction between killing and simply omitting life-sustaining treatment to let the patient die has a long history and is well understood by most clinicians, there is an intermediate case that has generated confusion. If a therapy is once begun, its withdrawal would seem to be morally similar to not providing it in the first place, and yet, psychologically, it may feel to many health care providers much closer to actively doing something to the patient to cause the patient's death. The following case asks how we should assess the withdrawal of a treatment that was begun because it might be beneficial, but is now being removed because it is believed not to offer benefits that exceed the burdens.

CASE 46: Withholding Versus Withdrawing

Robert Miner is a 23-year-old male with cystic fibrosis who has received treatment for his condition since his birth. He is aware that the maximal life expectancy for cystic fibrosis patients is approximately 23 or 24 years. For the past six months, he has been greatly depressed. He has talked with a psychologist about the prognosis for his condition. He knows that unless something unusual occurs he will die within another year.

Nancy Mills is Mr. Miner's respiratory care practitioner. She has provided treatment for him over the past three years. She has watched him go downhill and has seen his will to live evaporate.

Having been the recipient of ventilation treatment, Mr. Miner one day calls his physician to inform her that he no longer wants to be ventilated. The physician writes the order to discontinue ventilation on Mr. Miner's chart and informs the respiratory care office of the new orders. She indicates that it is the psychologist's opinion that, although he is depressed, the depression is appropriate for his condition. He is mentally competent to make judgments to refuse treatment.

Ms. Mills is caught off guard by this new development. She wonders if she must stop the ventilation support for him. It is tantamount to killing a patient, and she has always felt a strong commitment to sustain life. It strikes her that the physician merely writes the order, but she is going to have to physically remove the apparatus from her patient's face. Will she be responsible for killing her patient? Had the physician simply not initiated the ventilator, that would be different, it seemed to her, but once it was started, how can the physician expect her to remove it?

The agony of realizing that her action of removing the ventilator will be the immediate cause of the death of her patient might well be traumatic for Ms. Mills. The psychological impact is in some way linked to the moral issues, but in some sense it must be kept separate. The first issue is whether removing a ventilator at the request of the competent adult patient is morally any different from not starting it in the first place. The question is whether it is an instance of active killing, which we have seen, at least until state laws are changed, is illegal and widely considered to be unethical, or is an instance of forgoing treatment, which is legal and widely considered to be ethical.

The law makes a clear distinction between withdrawing life-sustaining treatment and active killing, treating killing as illegal while withdrawing treatment at the competent patient's request is treated as not only legal, but required. One approach to the problem is to view the decisions from the perspective of what the informed consent doctrine requires. Patients cannot be treated without consent, as we saw in the cases of Chapter 5. The autonomous patient has a right to agree or refuse to agree to any medical intervention. Presumably, Mr. Miner did this when the ventilator was initiated. When he did, it presumably made sense, because it would offer a significant chance of benefit. Otherwise, it is hard to see why he would have agreed to it.

But no rational consent would be open–ended; no rational person would agree to the use of the ventilator for ever and ever until death just because it seems to make sense for a time. In fact, many clinicians are recognizing that time-limited trials of possibly beneficial therapies often are more reasonable than some open-ended commitment that might lead care givers to mistakenly believe that the patient's permission goes on forever.

In the use of a ventilator, therefore, it is often wise to specify for how long the treatment will be tried. If no time limit is specified, the only reasonable conclusion is that if the patient has the authority to give permission to try a treatment, he also has the right to withdraw the permission and stop the treatment. Once the consent is withdrawn, what else can the provider do but take the treatment away?

In addition to the moral basis for removing such treatments, a pragmatic argument has been given for this approach. If the rule were that once an authorization for treatment were given it could not be withdrawn, there would be a strong incentive to not try an intervention unless one were very sure it would work. It seems irrational to avoid trying possibly effective life-prolonging interventions unless they were sure to succeed. The alternative is to permit patients or their surrogates to withdraw permission once the trial treatment is found wanting.

While the consent doctrine can force a provider to stop a treatment just the way it can force the provider not to begin, it can never force the provider to actively kill. From the point of view of the consent doctrine, withdrawing treatment is much more like withholding it than it is like active killing.

That, of course, does not deal with the very real psychological feeling that a respiratory care practitioner might have if she were forced by a physician to withdraw the ventilator knowing that the effect would be the death of her patient. For this reason, it is sometimes argued that physicians should not give such orders to other members of the health care team. If a treatment is to be withdrawn, the physician should strongly consider assuming the responsibility for the physical act of withdrawing the treatment rather than leaving that to other members of the team who may not have been directly involved with the patient when the decision was made. What should Ms. Mills do if she gets such an order? Should she be expected to do the actual removal of the ventilator or should she insist that the physician take that responsibility?

DIRECT VERSUS INDIRECT KILLING

The distinction between active killing and forgoing treatment is sometimes confused with another distinction that has become important in deciding whether it is morally wrong to kill another human being. Roman Catholic moral theology has long distinguished between directly intended evil and evil that is not intended. Theologians within this tradition (and many people in the secular world as well) have held that there are certain evils that are intrinsically wrong (such as killing an innocent person) and that it is always wrong directly to intend such evils. They have long recognized, however, that sometimes what they consider to be evil may occur even though it is not intended. Sometimes the one causing the evil may have no reasonable way of knowing that the evil would result, as when a health professional produces a fatal anaphylactic reaction by giving penicillin to a patient who is not suspected to be allergic. Surely, there is a sense in which the one who gave the unexpectedly dangerous drug killed the patient, and yet, just as certainly, the death was not intended. The health provider would have done anything to avoid the death, if only he had known. These "killings" are active killings, yet they are unintended; they are sometimes called indirect killings.

A more complicated case involves situations in which the evil is anticipated, but not desired. Some drugs are known to have undesirable side effects so that the health provider knows she is taking a risk by administering the drug. In some cases she may even know for sure that the side effect will occur, but consider the effect worth it. It may be known that giving an antihistamine will make the patient drowsy, but that, on balance, the antihistamine will benefit the patient. If it is given, we would not say that the provider intended to make the patient drowsy; rather, it was foreseen, unavoidable, though not intended.

Likewise, Catholic theologians have held that something as evil as a death may be morally tolerable if it is unintended, even if it is foreseen. If the patient dies from respiratory depression resulting from a heavy narcotic dose given to control pain, the death can be called an indirect killing, that is, one that, even though foreseen, is not intended.

Those who accept this distinction between direct and indirectly intended killing hold that, even though direct killings are never acceptable, under certain circumstances indirect killings are morally acceptable. To be acceptable, the evil must not be intended. Also, the good that is done, such as the relieving of pain, must be at least as great as the evil. Finally, the evil cannot be a means to the good end.[5]

Thus, according to Catholics, who believe that abortion is evil, it is unacceptable to abort a fetus to produce the "good" of relieving a pregnant woman's anxiety because the evil—the abortion—would be the means to the good. However, it might be acceptable to remove a cancerous uterus even if the woman with the cancer happened to be pregnant at the time. In the case of the cancer, the death of the fetus would not be a means to removing the cancer; it would be a foreseen, but unintended, side effect. In some cases, the harmful side effect for the fetus might not even be foreseen, as in cases in which a woman does not know that she is pregnant.

In caring for terminally ill patients, sometimes a health care worker may actively kill a patient by an intervention in which the death is foreseen, but unintended. In the following case, the issue is whether the fact that the death was not intended makes a moral difference.

CASE 47: Unintended, but Foreseen, Killing with an Overdose

This is one of many hospital admissions for a 60-year-old man with chronic obstructive pulmonary disease (COPD), who has smoked four packs of cigarettes a day for 40 years. On his last admission six months ago, diagnostic studies revealed advanced bronchogenic carcinoma. Given the patient's clinical picture of severe breathlessness, extreme pain, and low blood pressure, he is considered terminal. The nursing staff is quite concerned about the patient's moaning and pleading for "pain killers." Because of his deteriorating condition and history of lung disease, the PA is reluctant to order any narcotics and recommends nonnarcotic analgesics to be given.

As a last resort, the nursing staff summoned the attending physician, who prescribes a strong narcotic for injection. Within one hour of receiving the medication, the patient's breathing ceased, and he was pronounced dead.

During the next morning's rounds, the PA, who is visibly upset, asked for a private meeting with the physician. He says, "I don't understand your rationale for giving that patient such a strong narcotic. With his history of COPD, he was bound to die. It's like that shot killed him, and it's wrong to kill." The physician posed the question, "Is it right to let a patient suffer? Certainly the nonnarcotic analgesic could not relieve his unrelenting pain." The physician further defended the use of the narcotic on the grounds that the patient was in severe pain, and the purpose of the narcotic was to provide relief of pain. The physician recorded on the death certificate that the patient died as a result of his terminal conditions of COPD and lung cancer.

The death seems causally related to the administration of the narcotic, which is known to produce respiratory depression. For a patient in respiratory distress, it is not unexpected that further suppression of respiration would occur when the narcotic was administered. The first question to address is what the intention of the physician was and whether the intention matters morally in deciding whether he did wrong when he administered the narcotic. One possibility is that he simply intended to kill the patient in order to relieve his suffering. As we saw in an earlier case, had that been his intention, he certainly would be guilty of an illegal act, and most people seem to have concluded that such intentional, active killing of the patient is morally wrong as well.

But it might also be that his real intention was only to relieve the pain by whatever means was available and effective. If that were his intention, he would try to titrate the dose of the narcotic to avoid killing the patient. But suppose he realizes that he is approaching dangerously close to the point at which respiration would be fully suppressed. If he believes that approaching that point is necessary to achieve the intended goal of controlling pain, is the physician doing a moral wrong that is comparable to intended killing? Is a foreseen, but unintended, evil morally equivalent to an intended one?

Catholic theology insists that such risk of unintended, but foreseen, evil is tolerable. The *Ethical and Religious Directives* for Catholic Health Facilities state their position as follows: "It is not euthanasia to give a dying person sedatives and analgesics for the alleviation of pain, when such a measure is judged necessary, even though they may deprive the patient of the use of reason, or shorten his life."[6]

Other groups, however, dispute this conclusion. They might take the more liberal stance discussed in the previous case that holds that even active, intended killing for mercy (what the *Directives* called "euthanasia") is acceptable provided that all things considered it is the only way to relieve the suffering and does more good than harm. Others, more conservative, take a position that may be similar to the PA in this case. They hold that active, intended mercy killing is morally wrong, but that it is just as wrong to give the drug if the death will be foreseen even if it is not intended. A death is a death, according to this view.

Some who take that position emphasize that we must distinguish between the assessment of the moral blameworthiness of the actor and the moral rightness of the act. They might acknowledge that intention is important in assessing the character of the actor and conclude that it is a much worse moral character who intends the death compared to one who merely foresees that the death is a possibility while relief of pain is his sincere intention. Those who reject the distinction between direct and indirect (intended and foreseen) killing, however, say that when we are assessing the act itself, the same effect occurs regardless of the intention. If it is wrong to intend the death, it is just as wrong to act in such a way that one foresees the death will result, even though that is not the direct intention. The PA seems to take a position like this while the physician is either directly intending the death or, more likely, indirectly causing the death that he foresees but does not intend.

This is relevant to the related problem of what the physician should say on the death certificate. If administering this dose of narcotic analgesia is the moral equivalent of intending the death of the patient, then it makes sense to give the narcotic as the immediate cause of the death and to mention it on the death certificate, perhaps listing cancer as an underlying or secondary cause. If, however, lack of intention justifies treating such deaths as morally different (even if they are foreseen), then perhaps we should view the cancer as the cause of death rather than the narcotic. Many defenders of the distinction between intended and foreseen effects claim that interventions in which death is not intended should not be viewed as "causing" the death. Since these rather esoteric distinctions can lead to confusion and perhaps hide controversial behaviors (for example, if the physician fails to disclose that the narcotic contributed to the death), some people are now advocating that these contributing factors to a death should be reported even if they are not considered the cause of the death. If the physician is convinced that administering the narcotic was not the cause of the death because the death was not directly intended, he should be willing to defend his position publicly.

JUSTIFIABLE OMISSIONS

The last three cases have suggested that for one reason or another many people believe that active killings are morally unacceptable, at least if they are directly intended. The distinction between active killing and omitting treatment (sometimes referred to as the commission-omission distinction or the active-passive distinction) has grown to great importance in the debate over the care of the terminally ill. That is why it has been so important to figure out whether withdrawing a treatment is more like withholding it or more like active killing. Even if some treatments may justifiably be omitted, clearly not all can. The next case raises the issue of what is necessary to justify omission of treatment. In particular, are there certain kinds of treatments that can be forgone even though others never can be or is the criterion for justifying an omission based on assessment of benefit and harm? The next case poses the issue.

CASE 48: When Physical Therapy Is Too Great a Burden

Virginia Danson, a therapist at the Los Angeles Hospital Center, described a dilemma that she encountered frequently when she was working in acute care.

"Lots of times you feel that the patients are just too medically ill to begin rigorous treatment. Like when you see a lot of cancer patients who are dying and cannot really undergo as vigorous a treatment program as the physician recommends.

"For example, I worked with a gentleman who had cancer metastasis to the spinal cord. Basically, he was a paraplegic. They were pushing me to do the regular program for a spinal cord injury patient with him. It was like he just couldn't do it. He'd perspire, his blood pressure would go up, his heart rate would increase—you knew that he was really working at it. I would constantly complain to the doctor, and the doctor would ask, "How much can he bench press now?" or "Can he do his own transfers?" I would say, "He can't lift that much weight. And then I would get the dickens and the doctor would insist that I keep pushing him. The patient was only 42 but he was in an awful lot of pain."

Both secular and religious sources acknowledge that some treatments are so "extraordinary" that they are expendable.[7] We often think of high-technology treatments such as ventilators, dialysis machines, chemotherapy, or major surgery as treatments that might be expendable because they are "extraordinary." But that seems to assume that a treatment is considered extraordinary because it is statistically unusual or technologically complex.

Those who traditionally used the term *extraordinary* did not really have in mind the unusualness or complexity of the treatment. After all, it does not make much sense to consider a treatment expendable simply because it is unusual or complex. Something may be very unusual, but just right for a patient with an unusual condition. It may be high tech, but still very beneficial. The authorities that used to speak of extraordinary means of treatment now have tended to abandon that language because of this confusion. Instead, they make clear that treatments are morally expendable or required based on consideration of the benefits and burdens. If the benefits exceed the burdens, then the treatment is acceptable; if they do not, then it makes no sense to require it. This notion of the relative amount of benefits and burdens is now generally referred to as the *principle of proportionality*.[8] If the burdens equal or exceed the benefits, then there is no moral necessity to provide the treatment.

One remaining area of controversy is how the benefits and burdens are assessed. While some have traditionally believed that the benefits and the burdens can best be known by the physician, more recent commentaries have emphasized the subjective nature of these assessments. Hence, they have stressed that the physician has no special expertise in deciding whether an effect is a benefit and, if so, how beneficial it is. Likewise, the physician cannot have any special knowledge in deciding whether an effect is a harm, and, if so, how harmful.

Applying this reasoning to our case, how would Virginia Danson, the therapist, go about deciding whether the weight lifting and other exercises favored by the physician are morally necessary? Under the older idea in which the benefits and harms were believed to be determined based on medical expertise, the physician would be the one who would make the judgment. But if these assessments are subjective, then, according to the President's Commission, they should be assessed according to the patient's point of view.[9]

It is clear that the therapist believes that the exercises offer substantial burdens compared to the benefits. Should the therapist try to persuade the physician of this, or should it be left to the patient to determine?

VOLUNTARY AND INVOLUNTARY KILLING

In the previous cases we have seen that there is room for disagreement over whether some patients would be better off if they were dead. Those who focus exclusively on consequences would, logically, favor killing (or at least forgoing treatment) if they believed that the patient would be better off. On the other hand, those who accept that there is something inherently wrong with killing might continue to oppose active, direct killing even if they accepted the legitimacy of withholding or withdrawing treatment. There is one additional ethical principle that needs to be factored in. Especially if the decisions about what counts as a benefit or a harm are subjective, there may be good reasons to give moral weight to the autonomous choices of patients when it comes to deciding about whether to forgo life-sustaining treatment. In the following case, we shall explore the role of the autonomous choice of the patient in such decisions.

CASE 49: Assisting in a Suicide

Alice Simmons is a 44-year-old physician who is hospitalized for an acute relapse of her multiple sclerosis. She is depressed and angry as this is her third admission in the last 12 months, and her remissions are less complete. It is clear to her that her disease is accelerating and that it will not be too long before she will be unable to care for herself.

Dr. Simmons has always been a very independent person, and she has difficulty accepting the probability of her handicapped status. She believes that life would not be worth living if she could not continue to practice her profession and care for herself as she has done for so many years. She has expressed this sentiment to her family, friends, and professional colleagues.

Currently, Dr. Simmons is having great difficulty with ambulation, she is experiencing severe migraine headaches, and her ability to concentrate is significantly diminished. She is confined to her bed and placed on IV therapy to compensate for her refusal to eat.

Drew Douglas is a medical technologist who has known Dr. Simmons for many years. He has always liked and respected her and has felt personally hurt by her deteriorating condition. He has taken extended time to stay and visit with Dr. Simmons each time he was called upon to perform a venipuncture to obtain samples for the laboratory.

Mr. Douglas is well aware of Dr. Simmons' beliefs about her life. While he feels strongly that all persons have the right to determine the time to end their life, he does not believe that he could cooperate in the process. He is pulled between these two beliefs when Dr. Simmons asks that he leave a clean syringe for her.

Mr. Douglas thinks that Dr. Simmons will use the syringe to inject herself with some medication that she might obtain or that she might even attempt to inject air into her IV tubes. Does her wish to end her life justify this request? Would he be a participant to killing her? Can there be any basis for him to honor her request?

There is increasing controversy over the role of health professionals in assisting patients in bringing about their deaths. Physician killing on the persistent request of a competent patient is widely practiced in the Netherlands even though it technically remains illegal.[10] Legislative efforts are underway in several states that would legalize physician efforts to end a dying patient's life actively and intentionally.[11] One feature of these efforts, both in the Netherlands and in the United States, is that, if a physician is authorized to kill patients for a merciful motive, the plans carefully restrict such killing to patients who have made a voluntary request while they are mentally competent and, hence, able to make substantially autonomous choices.

The issue here is whether Dr. Simmons' request is voluntary, and, if so, whether that is a sufficient reason to judge Mr. Douglas's cooperation as ethically acceptable. First, is Dr. Simmons making a voluntary choice? If so, she would have to have the mental capacity to understand the nature of her choice and be substantially free from internal and external forces that would make her choice involuntary. Is she a substantially autonomous agent? What do you make of the claim that she is "depressed and angry"? Is that enough to make her incompetent to make a voluntary choice?

Assuming that she is substantially autonomous in her choice, does the principle of autonomy provide a moral basis for overcoming our general reluctance to cooperate in active killing of another human being or does the moral prohibition on killing, insofar as there is one, carry over to cases in which the patient has made a conscious, voluntary choice to end her life?

There is one final issue that needs to be addressed. Even if we conclude that Dr. Simmons has the right to kill herself, it does not necessarily follow that Mr. Douglas, as a medical technologist, has the moral right to cooperate by providing the syringe. Some would argue that even if, in theory, active mercy killing and suicide are legitimate, health professionals ought not be involved. They maintain that there is something about the role of being a health professional that is incompatible with killing even at the request of the patient and even if the killing is done for mercy. Is the fact that the patient in this case happens to be a physician relevant? If Mr. Douglas should give the syringe to Dr. Simmons, should he also give it to other patients who ask under similar circumstances?

The principles of avoidance of killing and autonomy seem to pull us in different directions in this case. To resolve the matter, we may have to appeal to our general theory of how to resolve conflict among principles. Does one of the two deserve priority such that it is ranked above the other permitting a ready formula for resolving the conflict? Or do both deserve consideration so that they are "balanced against each other" or in some other way combined to reach a final answer to the question of what Mr. Douglas's duty is?

This problem of conflict among the major principles of bioethics arises in many areas of health care ethics. In Part III we will look at some of those areas to see how the principles can be integrated to resolve potential conflicts.

ENDNOTES

1. John Rawls, "Two Concepts of Rules," *The Philosophical Review*, Vol. 44 (1955), pp. 3-32; David Lyons, *Forms and Limits of Utilitarianism* (Oxford: Oxford University Press, 1965); Paul Ramsey, *Deeds and Rules in Christian Ethics* (New York: Scribners, 1967); Richard B. Brandt, "Toward a Credible Form of Utilitarianism," in *Contemporary Utilitarianism*, ed. Michael D. Bayles (Garden City, NY: Doubleday, Company, 1968), pp. 143-186.
2. Ramsey, *Deeds and Rules in Christian Ethics.*
3. For example, see Immanuel Kant, *Groundwork of the Metaphysic of Morals*, trans. H. J. Paton. (New York: Harper and Row, 1964).
4. For a development of this view, see Robert M. Veatch, *A Theory of Medical Ethics* (New York: Basic Books, 1981), pp. 227ff.

5. Richard A. McCormick and Paul Ramsey, eds., *Doing Evil to Achieve Good: Moral Choice in Conflict Situations* (Chicago: Loyola University Press, 1978); Charles E. Curran, "Roman Catholicism," *Encyclopedia of Bioethics*, Vol. 4, ed. Warren T. Reich (New York: The Free Press, 1978), pp. 1522-1534; for secular treatments of the indirect or double-effect doctrine, see Philippa Foot, "The Problem of Abortion and the Doctrine of the Double Effect," *Oxford Review*, Vol. 5 (1967), pp. 5-15; Glenn C. Graber, "Some Questions About Double Effect," *Ethics in Science and Medicine*, Vol. 6, no. 1 (1979), pp. 65-84.
6. United States Catholic Conference, Department of Health Affairs, *Ethical and Religious Directives for Catholic Health Facilities* (Washington, DC: USCC, 1971).
7. Pope Pius XII, "The Prolongation of Life: An Address of Pope Pius XII to an International Congress of Anesthesiologists," *The Pope Speaks*, Vol. 4 (Spring 1958), pp. 393-398; President's Commission for the Study of Ethical Problems in Medicine and Biomedical and Behavioral Research, *Deciding to Forego Life-Sustaining Treatment: Ethical, Medical, and Legal Issues in Treatment Decisions* (Washington, DC: U.S. Government Printing Office, 1983).
8. Sacred Congregation for the Doctrine of the Faith, *Declaration on Euthanasia* (Rome: The Sacred Congregation, May 5, 1980; compare with the President's Commission, *Deciding to Forego Life-Sustaining Treatment*, p. 88.
9. Ibid.
10. Paul J. Van Der Mass, Johannes J. M. Van Delden, Loes Pijnenborg, and Casper W. N. Looman, "Euthanasia and Other Medical Decisions Concerning the End of Life," *The Lancet*, Vol. 338 (September 14, 1991), pp. 669-674.
11. Albert R. Jonsen, "Initiative 119: What Is at Stake?" *Commonweal*, Vol. 118, no. 14 (August 9, 1991), Suppl., pp. 466-469.

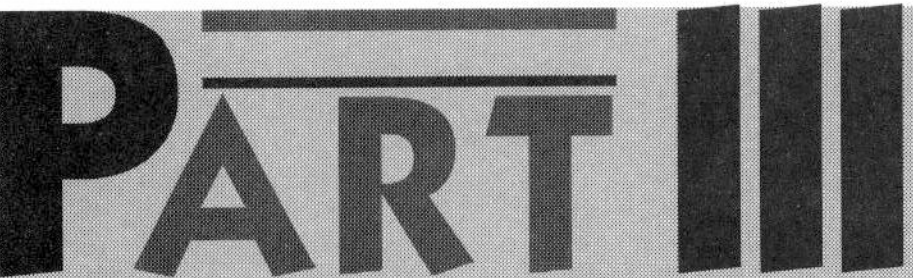

PART III

SPECIAL PROBLEM AREAS

CHAPTER 9

Abortion, Sterilization, and Contraception

One of the areas that has traditionally generated controversy in health care ethics is the set of problems surrounding obstetrics: abortion, sterilization, and contraception. All the general moral themes represented by the principles discussed in Part II arise, but they do so in a dramatic and often emotionally charged setting. Moreover, these issues of obstetrical ethics pose a different kind of question: To whom do the basic principles of biomedical ethics apply? We need to determine, for example, whether a principle such as avoiding killing applies to fetuses or to humans only after they are born. If it applies to fetuses, then we need to determine whether it applies to all fetuses or only to those with certain properties such as those with consciousness, the ability to move in a way perceived by the pregnant woman (quickening), or the ability to survive independently outside the womb. These issues also present a complex overlay of religious and philosophical notions about the duties and expectations of marriage, the role of natural law, and the role of the state in controlling intimate, personal choices. The first group of cases examines the ethics of abortion and the role of the allied health professional in abortions performed in a health care institution.

ABORTION

Perhaps the most controversial and intractable issue in health care ethics is abortion.[1] The underlying issue is what moral status and moral claims should be attributed to fetuses after conception has taken place and prior to birth. Do the normal moral principles such as beneficence and avoiding killing apply and, if not, why not?

What is at stake is nothing less than the moral standing of the fetus. If the fetus is considered nothing more than a part of the pregnant woman's body, then there is little reason to doubt that she can do whatever she pleases with it including removing it. On the other hand, if the fetus is considered to have the moral status of an independent human being with full moral standing, then the full range of principles we have been examining in this volume would apply to actions taken toward it. Not only would there be a *prima facie* duty to benefit and avoid harm, but there would also be a duty to keep promises made, to provide a just share of resources, and to avoid killing.

The most conservative position holds that the embryo has the full standing of other human beings from the moment of conception. The reason must be that at that time the embryo already has whatever is necessary to give it such standing. That might be the unique genetic composition or the genetic potential to develop certain features thought necessary to be treated as having this full standing. These features might be certain capacities for brain function or circulation and respiration.

Increasingly, controversy is emerging over exactly what gives this standing. For example, some have suggested that the genetic code may not actually be fixed exactly at the moment of conception, but may be capable of variation for some days thereafter. One Catholic bioethicist has suggested that the development of the so-called primitive streak signals the point at which a unique individual is established.[2] Others who are traditionally conservative have identified the latest point at which twinning can take place.[3] Still others may emphasize the development of more complex brain functions, but hold that what is critical is the potential for these functions as signaled by the presence of the genetic information that will be necessary for their expression.

Others, more liberal on the ethics of abortion, believe that some other functions, such as neurological integration, quickening, or the development of capacity for consciousness, must actually have appeared before the fetus has full moral standing. Of course, no one denies that from the moment of conception the embryo is made up of human cells. In that sense the tissues are "human." What is at stake is whether those tissues have moral claims against the rest of the human community. Some who hold these more liberal views would readily acknowledge that prior to the appearance of the feature they consider critical for full standing, there is some intermediate or lesser claim. Just as one might have an ethical duty to show respect for a human corpse after the death of an individual, so there might be a similar obligation to treat early embryos and fetuses with a certain degree of respect. What is the matter of real controversy is whether full equality of moral claims comes from the moment of conception or at some later time. In theory one might identify that moment even after birth. Some extreme commentators might hold, for example, that a newborn infant still lacks the key feature (such as the ability to reason or use language) that would give it a full claim against the human community. Most, however, recognize that at least by birth this full moral standing is present. The real controversy is whether it arises at conception or some later time and precisely what it is that is responsible for this standing.

Different reasons given for abortion raise these issues in different ways. For example, if someone proposed to abort a fetus because of a genetic abnormality, what would be at stake would be whether the key genetic characteristics are nevertheless present. Abortions proposed for other reasons, such as the health of the pregnant woman, rape, or socio-economic reasons, would require some argument supporting the abortion, even though the fetus presumably is genetically intact. The following cases all look at abortions for commonly proposed reasons.

1. Abortion for Genetic Reasons

One of the most commonly offered reasons for abortion is that the fetus has some genetic abnormality that justifies the abortion. This can happen on two different grounds. First, in some extreme cases the fetus might not have the genetic makeup considered essential for life. More often, the fetus unarguably has sufficient genetic material to live, at least for some time, but still has enough of a genetic problem that some might consider abortion justifiable. What is striking here is that the parents may, in general, be eager for a child. If they abort they will be deciding that this child is so compromised that the genetic problem warrants the abortion. Allied health personnel working in facilities that do abortions face the question of whether they will cooperate in such abortions. Others working in genetic counseling and prenatal diagnosis facilities will also. The following case illustrates the problem.

CASE 50: Aborting for a Serious Genetic Disorder

James Blackwell is a physical therapist working in County Hospital. He has a patient, Tim Honeycut, who lives in Kentucky, but comes to the city weekly for physical therapy treatment. Tim, who is 9 years old, has Duchenne muscular dystrophy, a genetic disorder that leaves victims chair-ridden by the age of 12 and dead by age 20. It is also associated with mental retardation. Tim's condition is terminal.

Mr. Blackwell is called into a conference with two physicians and Tim's parents, Mr. and Mrs. Honeycut. During the conference, it is disclosed that Mrs. Honeycut is pregnant again. Her obstetrician has said she is at about 18 weeks. It is certain through prenatal diagnosis that the child, if delivered to full term, will be born with the same disorder. James Blackwell was already aware that the Honeycuts had another child, Jack, who died three years ago from the same condition.

It becomes quite obvious to James Blackwell that the Honeycuts do not have the educational background to comprehend and understand the condition with which they and their children are afflicted. James Blackwell, like the other members of the team who are present, is asked to assist the physicians in convincing the Honeycuts to abort the fetus even though the pregnancy is quite advanced. Mr. Blackwell is torn by this request. Should he try to persuade the Honeycuts to seek an abortion?

There are at least two questions raised by this case. The first is substantive: Is it legitimate to abort a fetus because it is known to have the serious genetic disease, Duchenne muscular dystrophy? The second is more procedural: Should Mr. Blackwell cooperate in the effort to persuade the Honeycuts? Clearly, the two are linked, but separate, issues.

Serious genetic disorder is one of the reasons for abortion that has been found plausible even among those who object to abortion for more vague social and psychological reasons. The other "hard-core" reasons include rape, which will be discussed in Case 52, and incest, as well as the life of the pregnant woman.

This is a particularly serious genetic affliction. It will result in premature death and requires treatment during the period the child is alive. Yet terminating the pregnancy would involve active and direct killing, something those who oppose abortion would find unacceptable. Even if they accept the moral legitimacy of forgoing life support (as discussed in the cases in Chapter 8), they would not agree to active, direct killing even if it would spare the child certain suffering before it died. Only if ending this pregnancy were somehow morally different from killing a postnatal human would those who object to mercy killing agree to abortion. What reasons, if any, can be given for this difference? If the woman is now 18 weeks pregnant, the fetus is active and approaching the time when brain development is substantial and the fetus is viable to survive outside the womb. What is the relevance, if any, of these factors to the decision about aborting?

Mr. Blackwell must first decide whether he considers the abortion plausible. Then he has to address the difficult question of whether he should cooperate with the project of persuading the Honeycuts to abort. Assume first that he agrees that the abortion is defensible and the wise thing to do. Is it acceptable for a health care provider to try to persuade a patient to follow one moral course or another? On the one hand, he is pledged to do what he believes will benefit his patient. Even if we can determine whether his patient is the pregnant woman, the fetus, the afflicted child, or the entire family, he still might conclude that it is in his patient's interest to abort. Hippocratic ethics that mandate doing whatever is in the patient's interest would appear to favor the persuasion. In fact, extreme Hippocratic ethics, which will do anything to produce what the health provider believes will benefit the patient, might even favor lying to the patient or tricking her in order to get her to do what the provider feels will benefit her. But non-Hippocratic ethics favor leaving moral and other value choices more to patients. The principle of autonomy would support such a strategy, but autonomy does not require that a health provider participate in plans chosen by patients when the provider finds them unacceptable. Should Mr. Blackwell resist the strategy of persuasion in favor of one that is more neutrally informative? Are there some procedures in medicine about which providers ought not to be neutral?

This poses the question of how Mr. Blackwell should respond if he finds the abortion of a fetus with muscular dystrophy morally unacceptable. One possibility is that he could conscientiously refuse to participate. Health providers are generally considered to have such a right. That, however, would simply mean that Mrs. Honeycut would be subjected to persuasion from the rest of the cooperating team members without the offsetting presence of one who was not sympathetic. If he finds the abortion morally repulsive, is there anything more he can do other than refuse to participate?

There is still another complication here. It is possible that not all of the family will agree on what should be done. If several of the family members have differing views from that of the patient regarding the choice to be made, Mr. Blackwell would be in a position of supporting or contributing to internal family conflict if he were to decide to support one of the choice options and not the other. That would seem to be a reason supporting neutrality. However, if Mr. Blackwell's first job is to serve the patient, neutrality could be seen as an abandonment of the patient.

2. Abortion Following Maternal Trauma

Most abortions involve fetuses who themselves are not genetically afflicted. The reasons are based in the medical condition or desires of the pregnant woman and perhaps her husband. Abortions for rape have nothing to do with the genetic health of the fetus. If there is a reason to abort, it must be grounded in the lack of willingness of the woman to engage in intercourse. Abortions for socioeconomic reasons are based not in the fact that the woman was coerced, but rather in her desire not to become pregnant under her present circumstances.

Before turning to these cases, we will first examine a difficult case of a woman who suffered a head trauma while pregnant and was left in a condition that compromised the fetus' health and radically changed her own status.

CASE 51: Pregnant and Comatose: Is Abortion the Answer?

A teenage black female, age 16, was involved in an accident resulting in a severe head trauma leaving her in a coma from which she had only a slight chance of ever recovering. She was taken to University Hospital, the area's major tertiary care facility. During surgery, the patient was found to be two to three months pregnant. Family members were previously unaware of the pregnancy. The issue was should the doctors abort the fetus or keep it.

The family was informed. The patient's mother insisted that the pregnancy be continued. The health care team has another dilemma. If they were to maintain the pregnancy, they needed to provide adequate nutrition. Since she had a slight chance of recovering at least some degree of consciousness, some of the staff wanted to provide the total parenteral nutrition (TPN) in a way that would maximize the young woman's chances. That would involve 50 ml TPN with 20% fat.

Ginny Boston was the dietitian responsible for preparing the TPN. She knew that this formula would not be ideal for the fetus. An additional 500 calories would be necessary to support the fetus, but the physician responsible for the pregnant woman would not agree to such an increase. Moreover, Ms. Boston felt that if the young woman were to have the maximum chance of survival, she would do better if she were not pregnant. The fetus could be aborted, eliminating the conflict over the TPN formula as well as giving the woman the best chance of recovery. Ms. Boston knew the chance of her recovery was slim, but she had moral reservations about the effort to provide the nutrition at a level that would compromise the fetus' well-being. She thought they should either abort or provide the TPN appropriate for the fetus. If they chose the latter, they could attempt to maintain the fetus until it could be delivered prematurely by caesarean and agree to cease life support for the woman immediately after birth.

The technology is available now to maintain some severely compromised pregnant women long enough to attempt to carry the pregnancy to term.[4] If we knew the woman's own wishes, perhaps they could be seen as governing the choice,[5] but they are apparently unknown in this case.

Consider, first, the choice of the mother of the pregnant woman. It is widely held that the next of kin has the right to decide for or against life support for an incompetent patient such as this young woman. Normally, however, the next of kin would be expected to make a choice in the interest of the injured, incompetent patient. Here she seems to be deciding not on the basis of her daughter's interest, but on the basis of the interests of her possible future grandchild. Under those circumstances, should she insist on the TPN formulation that is best for the fetus regardless of the welfare of her child, or should she press for the therapy that serves her child's interest at the expense of her future grandchild? It is interesting to note that some state laws governing decisions to forgo life-sustaining treatment exclude the right of refusal of treatment in cases in which the patient is known to be pregnant.

On the other hand, if she desires to pursue the welfare of her daughter, she might have considered aborting the daughter's fetus to give her the best possible chance at recovery. If she did, she would be engaging in a choice for abortion for the health (and perhaps the life) of her daughter. It is often thought that if there is any possible justification for abortion, the life and health of the pregnant woman is the best one.

Ginny Boston is in the position of having to decide whether to jeopardize the fetus to encourage the maximum nutritional benefit for the young woman. If the choice made by the woman is to be supported by the nutritional formula ordered by the physician, Ms. Boston is put in an awkward position. The plan is really probably not the one that is best for the pregnant woman (aborting might accomplish this). On the other hand, the nutrition chosen is not best for the fetus either. If you were Ms. Boston, what would you choose? Would the remote chance of benefiting the woman justify aborting the fetus? Does the woman's mother have the right to jeopardize her daughter's interests in order to save the fetus? If so, does she have the right to authorize the TPN more fitting for the fetus' well-being?

3. Abortion Following a Rape

Another major reason offered for abortion is that the pregnant woman was raped and, therefore, did not consent to the risk of getting pregnant. In such a case, however, as contrasted to the previous ones, the fetus presumably is perfectly normal and not at significant medical risk. If the fetus is aborted, it is in order to serve the psychological well-being of the pregnant woman. Does the fact that the woman was exposed to pregnancy against her will justify aborting a presumably healthy fetus?

CASE 52: Reservations About Abortion Following a Rape

Jill Adams, a 22-year-old woman who was beaten and raped 10 weeks ago, presents to Dominic Vespucci, the physician assistant (PA) at the McLean Hospital clinic for evaluation of amenorrhea. McLean is a private, nonsectarian, voluntary facility. Other than a few fading bruises of the skin, the patient appeared in good physical condition. The laboratory test for pregnancy was confirmed, and, as the PA shared these results, the patient began to cry. She said, "I don't want to be pregnant, I'm a senior in college on financial aid, and I definitely don't want a baby by the guy who raped me. How can I get an abortion? What about these pills you can take for abortion?"

The PA, who is morally opposed to abortion, explains, "This is a big decision you're faced with. What you decide can affect you physically or mentally for the rest of your life. Before you make a decision, you might want to take some time to think this through. You've had a bad experience, but some good can come out of all this. One option you may consider is adoption. Why, you're in excellent physical condition and could have a healthy baby. There are so many couples looking for healthy babies to adopt. You could make someone very happy. Why don't I give you some literature on this and other options, and let's get together next week to talk about it."

In contrast to the two previous cases, neither the genetic status of the fetus nor the physical health of the pregnant woman provides any moral basis for aborting this pregnancy. Two reasons might be given. First, while Ms. Adams' physical health is not jeopardized by this pregnancy, her mental health might be. Surely, the trauma of the rape can be psychologically agonizing. Having the reminder of that horrid event during the rest of Ms. Adams' life could add to that trauma.

But if the woman's mental health is the basis for the abortion, some more information would be needed before Ms. Adams could make such a decision and Mr. Vespucci could consider trying to change her mind. First, they would have to have some understanding about just how much mental trauma is necessary to justify the abortion. Presumably, any unwanted pregnancy is traumatic. If just any mental disturbance justified the abortion, then any woman who was upset would be justified on these grounds.

The next case in this chapter looks at abortion for social and economic reasons. Is there a significant difference between abortion for the mental stress of a pregnancy following rape and abortion for the stress caused by social and economic reasons or for a woman who simply does not want to be pregnant? If the reasoning is based on mental health, is there some minimal level of psychological trauma that is necessary to make the abortion morally justified? For example, would a real risk of suicide be necessary as some conservatives on abortion would claim and, if so, what level of risk would be necessary? Or would any mental health risk be sufficient as more liberally inclined commentators would suggest? Would Mr. Vespucci's suggestion of adoption help abate some of this trauma, making the abortion less defensible?

Abortion following rape seems to command more sympathy than other cases involving similar levels of mental trauma. Could it be that there is some other reason beyond the psychological stress standing behind such intuitions? Some have argued that the morally special feature of rape is that in no conceivable way was the woman agreeing to take the risk of getting pregnant. Some philosophers have suggested that even if the fetus has the right to life in some strong sense, still a woman cannot be made to carry a pregnancy to term if she did not consent to the behavior that led to the pregnancy.[6] If it were technically possible, this could lead to removal of the fetus without jeopardizing its life. Until such a procedure is technically possible, defenders of abortion following rape say that the woman has a right to remove the "intruding" fetus even if that results in the death of the fetus.

More conservative critics of abortion reject this reasoning, pointing out that the end result is what, to them, is the evil of the death of the fetus. In the previous chapter, we discussed the Catholic doctrine of indirect or double-effect killing. This doctrine tolerates an evil if that evil is not intended and other conditions are met even if the evil is foreseen. They consider that this could justify removing a cancerous uterus even if the woman with the cancer happens to be pregnant as long as the death of the fetus is not the purpose of the removal of the uterus and the abortion is not a means to the desired end (which it would not be).

By contrast, if the woman claimed that she simply desired to be able to lead her life nonpregnant as she was prior to the rape, the abortion would be the means to her desired end, and according to Catholics and others who rely on the principle of indirect or double effect, the abortion would not be justified.

There is another issue in this case. Regardless of whether Ms. Adams decides the abortion is justified, Mr. Vespucci also faces an important moral choice. Were he in a federally funded facility under the Reagan and

Bush administrations he would have been under legal constraint that prohibited the discussion of abortion with clients.[7] That in itself is ethically controversial, but Mr. Vespucci is in a private voluntary facility. Discussing the abortion option is not, and never has been, prohibited. In fact, insofar as the informed consent doctrine requires presenting the alternatives that the patient would reasonably want to know about, there is good reason to believe that discussion of the abortion option is required morally and legally as part of the consent process. Either Mr. Vespucci or someone else would have that obligation.

Nevertheless, there are some procedures that would be such a dramatic violation of the conscience of the health provider that he or she would not be expected to discuss them and, in fact, might be expected to refuse to discuss them. For example, in some jurisdictions suicide is not illegal, and it could be considered a possible option for someone diagnosed as having a malignancy, yet it seems obvious that no health professional is required or expected to discuss the suicide option as part of the consent process for the treatment of the cancer. Likewise, most codes of ethics for health providers acknowledge that a provider is not required to be a party to a procedure that violates his or her conscience. The *Code of Ethics* of the American Academy of Physician Assistants does not specifically refer to such a right of its members to refuse to participate in actions that violate conscience, but it does contain provisions that could be interpreted by Mr. Vespucci to require that he not encourage the abortion. For example, it holds that the physician assistant "shall be committed to providing competent medical care, assuming as their primary responsibility the health, safety, welfare, and dignity of *all humans.*"[8] That provision could easily be interpreted by someone who opposed abortion as implying duties to protect the fetus. If someone else can take the case, part of the problem might be solved, but Mr. Vespucci may not have another PA to take the case and, even if he does, he may feel that even making a referral for what he considers to be murder to be unacceptable ethically. If Ms. Adams might be expected to want to discuss the abortion option more fully than she has to this point and Mr. Vespucci considers such conversations or referrals cooperation in a seriously immoral act, what can be done to resolve the conflict?

4. Abortion for Socioeconomic Reasons

In Case 52 we contrasted aborting because of the psychological trauma of a rape with more general psychological reasons grounded in the social and economic situation of the pregnant woman. The following case provides a context for examining the ethics of abortion for these more general socioeconomic reasons.

CASE 53: Should the Care Giver Suggest Aborting?

Yvonne Roberts is a 16-year-old mother who has a 2-year-old daughter, Leslie, who has Downs syndrome. This condition, which the genetic counselor has told her did not result from a translocation, is extremely rare in younger women—about 1 in 1,200. Because Ms. Roberts' daughter's condition was not the result of a translocation, her risk of having another such afflicted child is not any greater than any other woman's, less than 1 in a 100.

Ms. Roberts has just learned that she is six weeks pregnant. She lives at home with her mother, Mrs. Celo Roberts, and two other siblings in a two-bedroom apartment in federally subsidized housing. The counselor has told Ms. Roberts of the low risk that the Downs syndrome would recur in this pregnancy and that if she were worried, it could be determined via amniocentesis whether this had happened.

Felicia Cobert is a physical therapist who provides treatment for Yvonne Roberts' child who has Downs syndrome. Since she has been treating Leslie, Ms. Cobert has become very close to Leslie and her mother. Ms. Cobert believes that Ms. Roberts does not have the necessary economic or emotional resources to care for Leslie and a new infant, regardless of whether it is healthy.

At the same time, Ms. Cobert struggles with her tendency to become overly involved with her clients. After all, Ms. Cobert is not a counselor. Leslie, not Ms. Roberts, is Ms. Cobert's patient. Yet, Ms. Cobert just knows what is going to happen to Ms. Roberts if nothing is said to her. Should Ms. Cobert try to persuade Ms. Roberts to have an abortion?

It is easy to understand why Ms. Cobert might be concerned about the effect of another pregnancy on Yvonne Roberts and her family. If she is to work with her client to determine whether an abortion is appropriate here, she first needs to decide whether the social and economic conditions in which this family resides justifies terminating the pregnancy.

While Ms. Roberts has already borne a child suffering a serious genetic affliction, she is apparently only at slightly greater risk of having another child with Downs syndrome. Moreover, if she is really worried about this possibility, she could have an amniocentesis during the mid-trimester of her pregnancy and then make a decision about abortion. That would mean a later abortion, but would be an approach many women would choose if they were only worried about the risk of another afflicted infant.

Ms. Cobert is apparently not worried about this so much as the fact that this family is already under severe economic and emotional stress and could be further traumatized by another pregnancy, regardless of whether that pregnancy resulted in a healthy child. Ms. Cobert knows that many families in this situation would at least want to consider abortion. On the other hand, she knows that pregnancy is psychologically and socially important to many unwed adolescents. They would no sooner abort a pregnancy than place their children for adoption.

Ms. Cobert is a physical therapist, not a counselor. Yet she believes she knows something that could be relevant to the welfare of her patient (Leslie) as well as the rest of her family. If she feels the abortion would be justified, what are her options? Should she raise the issue with Yvonne Roberts, refer her to the obstetric department for further discussion, or simply let the matter drop? Are there other alternatives?

STERILIZATION

Another intervention that has traditionally raised moral controversy in biomedical ethics is sterilization. Designed to permanently prohibit fertility, it has run afoul of Catholics and others who apply natural law reasoning to matters of medical morality.[9] They hold that there are certain "natural ends" of human beings that are associated with certain bodily organs and tissues. They hold that one of the natural ends of the human is to procreate and that any directly intended interference with these functions violates the moral law.

Others, who may not share this natural law reasoning, also encounter moral problems related to sterilization. Low-income women have reported being pressured by health care professionals to consent to being sterilized out of a paternalistic concern by the providers that pregnancy would not be good for either the woman or her offspring. Other women, as in the following case, have reported finding it extremely difficult to convince physicians to sterilize them, especially if they were not considered old for child-bearing or had not already given birth to a number of children.[10]

CASE 54: Keeping Options Open: Is Sterilization Appropriate?

Mrs. Laura Simpson has come to have lunch with her close friend, Susan Hill, while at the hospital for her six-week checkup following the birth of her fourth child. Ms. Hill is a medical technologist working at the facility with personal and professional knowledge of Laura Simpson's situation.

During the course of lunch, Mrs. Simpson indicates her distress that her physician, Dr. James Sargent, has not agreed to her request for sterilization. While he agrees that she should not have additional children soon, she is fundamentally in good health. Each of her children was born within a 12- to 14-month period of each other, which accounts for her anemia, mild depression, and sense of foreboding about the future. The physician advises more attention to birth control.

Susan Hill is concerned that her friend is not receiving good medical advice. Her concern is based upon her knowledge that Laura Simpson is in an abusive relationship that she feels powerless to change. It is unlikely that birth control will be more effective in the future as her husband wants "a dozen kids." More important, she is concerned that Mrs. Simpson's prior atypical Pap smears are being ignored.

For the past two years, Laura Simpson has had Pap smears indicative of dysplasia. Under routine circumstances she could be a candidate for medical follow-up, and, given her history and personal life, a hysterectomy appears warranted. However, Dr. Sargent is loath to recommend or concur with Mrs. Simpson's request because of his personal beliefs concerning sterilization. It is his view that sterilization is inappropriate except in extreme circumstances. He does not define Mrs. Simpson's case as extreme.

Susan Hill is uncertain whether it is ethical for her to discuss Dr. Sargent's beliefs with her friend. She is further torn on the advisability of discussing the implication of the Pap smears, the anemia, and other indicators of health.

This case presents a complex combination of religious, medical, and personal issues for Ms. Hill. Focus first on the ethical issues about sterilization. What is the reason for Dr. Sargent's resistance to the sterilization? One possibility is that he opposes all sterilizations as a violation of the moral natural law. Surely, sterilization will permanently disrupt the reproductive function, considered by many, including many Catholics, to be a "primary end of marriage."

Nothing in the case indicated that Dr. Sargent was Catholic. In fact, if there is some medical reason related to the Pap smear to remove Mrs. Simpson's uterus, most proponents of Catholic moral theology would not object. They would consider the effect on her fertility to be an indirect effect, one not directly intended. Even if that effect could be foreseen, as surely it could be, a hysterectomy would be morally acceptable in these circumstances.

But there are other reasons why physicians and others have traditionally objected to sterilizations. Especially among Protestant and liberal, secular thinkers, there is virtue in keeping one's options open. Permanent loss of fertility has been seen as foreclosing options. Such objectors have a strong preference for temporary forms of birth control, as Dr. Sargent apparently did. Would the advantage of keeping options open justify Dr. Sargent's resistance to the sterilization in this case?

Ms. Hill also expresses concern about whether it is appropriate to discuss the alternatives and Dr. Sargent's views with her friend. While discussion of the physician's personal ethical views might normally be inappropriate, in this case those views seem to be having a direct bearing on Mrs. Simpson's treatment. Does that fact justify the discussion? What reasons would she have for resisting the discussion? Given the fact that Mrs. Simpson has expressed a clear desire for sterilization, would it be appropriate for Ms. Hill to suggest that Mrs. Simpson transfer to another physician more compatible with her views?

CONTRACEPTION

The third area of moral concern related to fertility and birth is contraception. Until the 1930s most of the major religious traditions had moral objections to efforts to control fertility through contraception. The techniques that were available were not very reliable and such efforts were seen as infringing on the traditional "duties of marriage" as well as furthering promiscuity in sexual relations.

In 1930 the Lambeth Conference signaled the willingness of the Anglican tradition to open the door cautiously to some fertility control. The other Protestant traditions soon followed,[11] but Catholic moral theology reinforced its traditional view that all sexual acts had to be open to procreation as well as expressing the unity of marriage.[12] The mainstream of Catholic thought accepted that the rhythm method of fertility control, which was considered "natural," might be acceptable, but no barrier methods were because they interfered with the natural ends of marriage. By the 1960s some Catholics began to consider this strong prohibition unnecessary, particularly becoming open to the use of the new oral contraceptives.[13] The majority of a papal commission considered such an opening acceptable, but with the papal encyclical *Humane Vitae,* a condemnation of all except so-called natural methods was reaffirmed.[14] Similar disputes arose in the Jewish tradition with the Jewish commitment to the duty to procreate in conflict with more liberal acceptance of self-determination regarding fertility.[15] There is increasing evidence that all people have underlying value commitments that will have influence on medical decisions. These will be manifest in decisions about birth control in which even those who are attempting to be fair and neutral may use language in ways that reflect their value commitments.[16]

As seen in the next case, allied health care providers may find themselves in positions in which they are to teach or counsel about fertility control.

CASE 55: Biased Counseling: Teaching About Birth Control

Margaret Evanson, a staff PA, was asked to conduct a one-hour session on contraceptive methods for patients attending the gynecology clinic. Being reared in a large Catholic family, Ms. Evanson had some biases and tended to emphasize those methods that she could morally support.

Ms. Evanson started off the presentation by saying, "You may find it interesting to know that the number of birth control methods approved for use in this country is smaller today than a decade ago. It could be that Americans are becoming more health conscious. We're beginning to learn that all of these unnatural products in our bodies can harm us. I'm sure that many of you have heard about the terrible effects of interuterine devices (IUDs), for example. Many women have suffered from these devices and other birth control methods, and some have lost their ability to bear children. I think that history has taught us that natural methods are the safest methods. Certainly all birth control methods have their strong points and weak points. And if we are very careful we can select those methods that do not place us at unnecessary risk. Now let us review in detail the various types ..."

Those who are more accepting of birth control are likely to accuse Ms. Evanson of being biased in her presentation. This matter of bias, however, is rather complex. Probably everything she said had a basis in fact. It was not that she was purposely saying untrue things about birth control. In fact, what she was saying probably could be supported by good scientific data. Some methods—high dose oral contraceptives and some IUDs--have been removed from the market because of their risks. Yet she seems to have selected the data she presented.

She may be in a position that is not as different from her colleagues as she might expect. Any health educator has a virtually infinite array of information that he or she may transmit. He or she must select those data that seem most interesting and important. Those selections must be made on the basis of one's beliefs and values about what is important. Every communication with a patient will be shaped in this way, at least to some extent.

Assuming this is true, what should Ms. Evanson have done? Assuming she strongly believes, based on her knowledge of the data and her sense of what is important, that artificial methods of birth control cause problems that are not worth the risks, how should she communicate her understanding to the patient?

A colleague of Ms. Evanson's who had strong feelings that oral contraceptives and other so-called artificial methods had benefits that far exceeded the risks is in a position that is more similar to Ms. Evanson's than many people realize. They also will have to choose from an infinite array of possible facts those that are worth communicating.

One response is to try to be "value neutral" in communicating with patients. That may be harder than it sounds. Since one cannot give "all" the facts, some will have to be selected. Words with shades of meaning will have to be communicated. Moreover, some health care providers may believe that some options are inherently so immoral that they simply cannot be presented in a cold, hard, value-neutral manner. Infanticide is a method of controlling family size that has been used by some cultures, and it is not unheard of in contemporary Western culture. Yet surely no health care provider would list among the methods available that one can always take the child after birth and kill it. Only those methods that are morally and legally plausible should be presented.

This raises a major problem for the allied health care provider. Can she simply refuse to participate in services for patients that violate her conscience? If so, will that not leave the educational task for matters like abortion, sterilization, and birth control to those who have not disqualified themselves, making the group systematically skewed toward a more accepting position? What are Ms. Evanson's options here? What are the options of her supervisor if Ms. Evanson fails to disqualify herself or if the one given the task appears to be giving an unusually favorable presentation of the methods of which Ms. Evanson disapproves?

ENDNOTES

1. For further discussion of the ethics of abortion, see Daniel Callahan, *Abortion: Law, Choice and Morality* (New York: Macmillan, 1970); Joel Feinberg, ed., *The Problem of Abortion* (Belmont, CA: Wadsworth, 1973); Michael D. Bayles, *Reproductive Ethics* (Englewood Cliffs, NJ: Prentice Hall, 1984); and John T. Noonan, *The Morality of Abortion: Legal and Historical Perspectives* (Cambridge, MA: Harvard University Press, 1970).
2. Richard A. McCormick, "Who or What Is the Preembryo?" *Kennedy Institute of Ethics Journal*, Vol. 1 (1991), pp. 1-15, esp. pp. 4, 9, 11-12.
3. A. Hellegers, "Fetal Development," *Theological Studies* 31 (March 1970), pp. 3-9.
4. William P. Dillon, Richard V. Lee, Michael J. Tronolone, Sharon Buckwald, and Ronald J. Foote, "Life Support and Maternal Brain Death During Pregnancy," *Journal of the American Medical Association*, Vol. 248 (September 2, 1982), pp. 1089-1091.
5. *In re A.C.*, 533 A.2d 611 (D.C. App. 1987).
6. Judith Jarvis Thomson, "A Defense of Abortion," *Philosophy and Public Affairs*, Vol. 1, no. 1 (Fall 1971), pp. 47-66.
7. M. Gregg Bloche, "The 'Gag Rule' Revisited: Physicians as Abortion Gatekeepers," *Law, Medicine and Health Care*, Vol. 20 (1992), pp. 392-402; Jeremy Sugarman and Madison Powers, "How the Doctor Got Gagged: The Disintegrating Right of Privacy in the Physician-Patient Relationship," *Journal of the American Medical Association*, Vol. 266 (1991), pp. 3323-3327.
8. American Academy of Physician Assistants, *Code of Ethics of the Physician Assistant Profession* (Alexandria, VA: AAPA, adopted 1983, amended 1985 House of Delegates).
9. Benedict M. Ashley and Kevin D. O'Rourke, *Healthcare Ethics: A Theological Analysis*, 3rd ed. (St. Louis: The Catholic Health Association of the United States, 1989).
10. Susan C. Scrimshaw and Bernard Pasquariella, "Obstacles to Sterilization in One Community," *Family Planning Perspectives*, Vol. 2 (1970), pp. 40-42.
11. Richard M. Fagley, *The Population Explosion and Christian Responsibility* (New York: Oxford University Press, 1960).
12. John T. Noonan, *Contraception: A History of Its Treatment by the Catholic Theologians and Canonists* (Cambridge, MA: Harvard University, 1966).
13. Daniel Callahan, ed., *The Catholic Case for Contraception* (New York: Macmillan, 1969).

14. Pope Paul VI, "Encyclical Letter on the Regulation of Births (July 25, 1968)," in *Medical Ethics: Sources of Catholic Teachings*, eds. Kevin D. O'Rourke and Philip Boyle (St. Louis: The Catholic Health Association of the United States, 1989), pp. 85-91.
15. David M. Feldman, *Birth Control in Jewish Law* (New York: New York University Press, 1968).
16. Robert M. Veatch, *Value-Freedom in Science and Technology* (Missoula, MT: Scholars Press, 1976).

CHAPTER 10

Genetics, Birth, and the Biological Revolution

In addition to the moral problems related to contraception, sterilization, and abortion, which were addressed in Chapter 9, there are emerging newer, more complex, ethical questions connected with the process of conception, prenatal development, and birth.[1] Some of these issues are related to the increasing importance of the science of genetics. For many years we have had a vague idea that certain diseases were inherited, but only recently have we had the precise knowledge and ability to determine the chances that a disease will be transmitted and to counsel the prospective parents about intervention alternatives.

The first level of such counseling involves assessing and informing parents whether a condition is inherited, and if so, how. It may now involve prenatal sampling of amniotic fluid or chorionic villa blood sampling that permits either chromosomal or biochemical determinations of whether a fetus already gestating is infected with a disease.[2] Other efforts are oriented toward genetic screening of larger populations at risk for conditions such as Tay Sachs disease so that individuals can be informed about whether they are at risk for conceiving an afflicted child and, if they are, what the chances are of child being affected.[3] When one shifts to mass screening, additional moral problems—confidentiality, record keeping, statistical morality—come into play.

More recently, the technologies related to in vitro fertilization—removing an egg from a woman and fertilizing it in the laboratory—have posed new and controversial problems.[4] Allied health personnel including lab technicians and physicians' assistants have found themselves in positions in which they are asked to manipulate human embryos, store them, freeze them, and even discard those not needed.

Once the technology to fertilize human eggs outside the woman's body is available, there is no technical reason why the fertilized egg needs to be returned to the woman from whom the egg was taken. Surrogate motherhood involves reimplanting the fertilized egg into some other woman either so that she may bear the child and continue to be its mother after the birth or so that she may bear the child in order to return him or her for parenting to the woman who supplied the egg.[5] In theory the egg could be obtained from one woman, gestated and delivered by a second, and parented by a third.

Still newer and more controversial is what is referred to as gene therapy or genetic engineering.[6] Efforts are under way to modify the actual genetic codes of patients suffering from genetic diseases. These have already been attempted to treat some conditions such as the enzyme deficiency, ADA deficiency, and research is developing rapidly to use similar technologies to treat other conditions. The first efforts are designed to modify somatic cells (so that only the treated individual and not his or her offspring will have the genetic material changed). Eventually, similar technologies will probably be used to modify reproductive cells (so that the genetic change will be transmitted to the offspring).

Ethical problems arise at many levels with these birth technologies. Perhaps the most fundamental issue is whether tampering with the genetic and birth processes is "playing God" in an unacceptable way. Such technologies have the potential to change the nature of the human species. While the species undoubtedly is already undergoing change, changes to date have been in a much slower, unplanned evolutionary fashion. The technologies under development have the potential for much more rapid change in the genetic character of the species as well as in the basic biological processes such as reproduction. The first question raised is thus whether such efforts extend beyond what humans should be permitted to do.

Even if one accepts the idea in principle of producing such fundamental changes, there will remain controversy over just which changes are ethically acceptable. This will, in turn, require judgments about what conditions in our species are unacceptable. Everyone might agree that a terrible disease like Lesch-Nyhan syndrome—incompatible with life of more than a few months and dreadfully painful while the infant is alive—is a condition worth changing if we can; however, the same technologies are likely to permit us to intervene to modify conditions less obviously unacceptable. Color-blindness, for example, might be amenable to some of these technologies. Even conceiving an embryo of an undesired sex can be diagnosed prenatally and is, in principle, subject to interventions. The question is, "Does such a condition justify genetic interventions?"

Many other moral problems arise with these technologies: problems of identifying unexpected paternity, notifying other family members of the diagnosis of a genetic anomaly, and conflicts among parties over custody of a child. The cases in this chapter raise many of these issues.

GENETIC COUNSELING

Increasingly, allied health professionals working in obstetrics departments and in genetic counseling services will be involved in communication with patients who are being counseled about the statistical risk of conceiving a child with a genetic anomaly.[7] This could involve a condition already present in a child, a parent, or some other member of the family. Or it could involve concern about a new genetic problem such as the risk of an older woman conceiving a child with trisomy 21 (Downs syndrome). The following two cases show how allied health personnel are involved in ethical problems of genetic counseling.

CASE 56: A Genetic Skeleton in the Family Closet?

Frank Goldfarb, a 23-year-old man, appeared at the Medical Records Department of a long-term care facility. This facility included skilled, intermediate, and long-term/custodial care, as well as residential accommodations for the elderly. The young man asked the medical records administrator for information about his maternal grandfather, who had lived at the facility for more than 20 years, when he was in his sixties and seventies, but had not died there. He had no information as to where or from what his grandfather had died and no one in his family would discuss the grandfather or what had happened to him. Mr. Goldfarb was generally aware from his memory of his grandfather that he acted strangely, had a difficult time remembering things, and, near death, did not even recognize his family members.

The young man was about to be married and was concerned about the mystery surrounding his grandfather's demise; he was especially interested in obtaining information relevant to genetic history, in view of his impending marriage. His mother had died of breast cancer three years previously at age 58, but Mr. Goldfarb had been concerned that before her death she had begun to show early signs of premature senility. He had no idea whether her condition was related to his grandfather's, but he was curious. He did not have an authorization form from his grandfather's next of kin (Mr. Goldfarb's uncle) to obtain information from the patient record, as the knowledgeable family members had closed ranks and refused to discuss the grandfather. State law and institutional policy required a signed authorization form from the next of kin to release information from the medical record of a deceased patient.

Mr. Goldfarb is concerned about the risk that he could be carrying genes that were somehow responsible for his grandfather's undisclosed illness. There is suspicion that his mother had the condition. If the problem were caused by a single gene that was dominant (and therefore caused the disease in all offspring inheriting it), Mr. Goldfarb should be concerned only if his mother had the problem. If she did, then there is a 50-50 chance he would have it as well. Mr. Goldfarb need not be concerned unless she also had the disease, but since she died rather early in life, there is no way to tell for sure whether she did. If it were caused by a single recessive gene, even if his mother inherited the gene from her father, Mr. Goldfarb would be at risk only if her husband also happened to be carrying the gene, a remote possibility unless the condition were very common.

There is also a possibility that his grandfather's condition was caused by a larger number of genes, some of which could have been transmitted through his mother to Mr. Goldfarb.

Given that Mr. Goldfarb knows relatively little about the problems his grandfather and mother suffered, he has some reason to inquire. The moral problem arises because medical information, particularly sensitive genetic information, is deemed confidential. Thus, the ethics of confidentiality, discussed in Chapter 7, comes into play.

It is not uncommon for families to want to keep information about family members with chronic illnesses, especially mental illnesses, hidden from outsiders. Since some such conditions have a genetic component, they must fear that if such knowledge were known, it would cast aspersions on them as well. The stigmatizing of individuals who have mental problems and even of those who have such problems in their families is well known.[8] Thus, the first issue raised by this case is whether the family is being fair with Mr. Goldfarb and other descendants by refusing to disclose the information about the grandfather. If such information is, in fact, stigmatizing, are they justified in keeping this information secret?

Assuming Mr. Goldfarb has some legitimate concern about his grandfather's genetic history, it seems that a good case can be made that those in the family who know the history or control the information should be willing to disclose it. Are there any reasons why it should not be disclosed, assuming that Mr. Goldfarb will be discrete in what he does with it?

If he does have a legitimate interest in the information, should the medical records or health information administrator be willing to disclose it? We saw in the discussion of confidentiality that health professionals generally are committed to protecting confidential information; it is part of their promise to patients in the establishment of the health professional-patient relation. Most ethical systems, however, acknowledge some exceptions. The Hippocratic tradition would permit breaking confidence whenever it was for the benefit of the patient. That seems unlikely here since their patient (the grandfather) is dead. However, conceivably one could argue that it would have been in the grandfather's interest to have his grandson informed about the genetic elements of his illness, if any.

The utilitarian tradition would permit exceptions whenever it serves the total good, taking into account not only the grandfather's interests, but also Mr. Goldfarb's (and his future wife's). Utilitarians, however, would also need to take into account the interests of the other relatives—those who are refusing to release the information. Would a utilitarian favor the release of records? Some utilitarians would actually base their judgment on the issue of what general practices will produce the most good. This approach is what in the introduction we called *rule-utilitarianism*. Would a general practice of releasing genetic information to relatives when they have an interest like that of Mr. Goldfarb be likely to do more harm or good in the long run?

Many ethical commentators on confidentiality, including the AMA,[9] are unwilling to support disclosures based either on the interest of the patient or the combined general social interests of all other parties. They are moving toward a narrowly defined exception clause to the confidentiality rule that would permit disclosure only when there is a serious threat of grave bodily harm to another party. Would such an exception clause apply in this case? Could Mr. Goldfarb's interest be construed as a serious threat of grave bodily harm?

In the case of the American Health Information Management Association *Code of Ethics*, it could be argued that there are conflicting ethical standards that relate to the Goldfarb case. On the one hand, in their official interpretation of their code, principle 1 requires that the health information professional should ensure that all patient-identifying information will be kept confidential, the strict interpretation of which would suggest that the health information administrator should keep the patient's records in confidence. At the same time, their interpretation of principle 9 holds that the health information professional should advocate policies that will result in the optimal use of patient records for the patient, institution, and the public. Since the patient is deceased, benefit to the public would certainly be included in the calculation in the Goldfarb case. As suggested in Chapter 7, professional codes can have internal inconsistencies or conflict with the codes of other professional groups or those of a particular institution.

CASE 57: Does Genetic Counseling Include Making Recommendations?

In an attempt to provide as much information as possible to clients needing to make decisions about their pregnancies, the Obstetrics and Gynecology Department of Springfield Hospital determined that the cytogenetic technologists should assist in the counseling process. Counseling teams were established with each team consisting of a physician, nurse, member of the clergy, and the technologist. The role of the cytogenetic technologist was to provide data about chromosomal and biochemical abnormalities, statistical probabilities, and evaluation techniques.

James Morison was a cytogenetic technologist who was joining such a counseling team. While courses in counseling had been included in Mr. Morison's educational program, this assignment was the first real experience that he had had in the counseling process. He is confronted almost immediately with the assessment of how to balance appropriately his role as a fact giver with his inclination to offer advice. It becomes clear that the facts are interpreted differently by each client and that he must assume more responsibility for interpretation of the information to the client.

When presented with information about the presence of an abnormality, some clients immediately opt for abortion, regardless of the severity of the problem. Other women insist on carrying to term babies that will be seriously deformed with little hope of a normal life. The technologist must find some way of assisting these women in making informed decisions.

For example, Mr. Morison's first case involved a 35-year-old married woman who was 18 weeks pregnant and had been diagnosed prenatally as carrying an infant with Downs syndrome. The woman was poorly educated and had a difficult time understanding the nature of the problem. She and her husband were living on a combined income that was barely above the poverty level. They were nonpracticing Catholics. She was told that the infant would have certain characteristic physical features. (She was shown several pictures of Downs syndrome children to help her understand.) She was also told that the boy—the prenatal diagnosis necessarily reveals the fetus' sex—would have some unknown degree of mental retardation, but would not suffer physically unless other problems arose that sometimes accompany

Downs syndrome. She was told that there was no medical cure for the underlying condition and that legally she could have an abortion. The child would probably require special education and other supports to learn to adjust to his life with this condition.

As a member of a team, not as a solo counselor, what is the technologist's responsibility? Do the physicians and clergy have greater responsibility for offering advice? How directive should the team be in determining the outcome of the pregnancy? Is the client only the woman or must her fetus be considered? What should the cytogenetic technologist do?

As was noted in the discussion in Chapter 1, it is extremely difficult, probably impossible, for an expert in a field to impart pure, "value-free" facts. Mr. Morison could have said a very large number of things about Downs syndrome and this woman's options. Some were very technical; some most people would consider trivial. Some involved options that the patient almost certainly would not choose, and even if she would, there would be moral problems had Mr. Morison suggested them. (For example, suicide is a possibility for this woman, but no one would really expect Mr. Morison to present it as a choice to consider).

Mr. Morison found that patients may have a hard time recognizing the value component in the communications. Yet every piece of the message can be phrased—perhaps must be phrased—so as to incline the patient hearing it to pursue a certain course. Saying that the child will have some degree of mental retardation, for example, will arouse certain anxieties. That could be followed with additional information that would tend to calm those anxieties—that counseling will be available, that the woman can meet with other parents who are successfully raising Downs syndrome children. It could also be followed with more threatening information—that many people rightly or wrongly will stigmatize their boy, that certain aspirations they have for their child may not be obtainable, and so forth.

One possibility is for Mr. Morison to yield to the other members of the health care team, but they are in essentially similar positions. They also will have to communicate messages that contain value judgments. The clergy member of the team quite clearly will have a religious moral framework upon which to draw, but the physician and Mr. Morison will also necessarily be drawing on some religious or secular framework. Can all the members of the team offer their personal opinions about what should be done, emphasizing that these are personal views based on religious and other beliefs and values? Or should they try to hide their personal opinions and insist that this woman make her own choices?

GENETIC SCREENING

Sometimes genetic counseling arises in the context of community-based genetic screening programs. These differ from the previous case in that the allied health person would be involved in a mass or group screening rather than one-on-one counseling. These efforts often take place in churches or community programs in which the professional staff really have no ongoing contact with the patients. Sometimes these programs have racial or ethnic implications complicating the counseling. For example, proposals to screen for sickle-cell anemia, a blood disease affecting primarily persons of African origin, raise issues of whether the purpose was to discourage fertility among this group. One major effort has been directed toward Tay Sachs within the Jewish community. Tay Sachs is a devastating disease that leads quickly to complete loss of bodily functions and death within a few months, but it is an autosomal recessive and carriers of the disease lead perfectly normal lives. The primary purposes of the screening are to discourage fertility when two people with the recessive gene marry or to identify and abort fetuses with the actual disease. Both discouraging fertility and facilitating abortion are morally controversial within the Jewish community.

CASE 58: Genetic Screening to Reduce Tay Sachs Disease

Deborah Schwartz has been actively involved in her synagogue since early childhood. This involvement has taken many forms, with one major area of emphasis involving programs of health promotion. As a laboratory professional she has encouraged and assisted in the organization of blood pressure screening, diabetes detection, cholesterol checks, and general fitness evaluations. As a result of her efforts, a significant level of health consciousness has developed among members of the congregation.

Following the unfortunate death of a young child with Tay Sachs disease, the community health committee of the synagogue voted to initiate a Tay Sachs screening program. This program was designed to offer testing to all pregnant women and all couples planning marriage. The discussions and vote on this program occurred while Ms. Schwartz was on vacation.

Upon learning of the plans for the screening program, Ms. Schwartz immediately began to raise questions. She learned that pregnant women with positive tests would be counseled to have abortions and engaged couples would be advised to avoid having children. Ms. Schwartz was philosophically against this component of the screening program.

With a personal family history of victims of the Holocaust, Deborah Schwartz was raised to believe in the sanctity of life and the need to preserve the Jewish faith through continual creation of new lives. This program was being developed in a manner that was the antithesis of her beliefs.

As a health professional, Ms. Schwartz supported the concept of all people knowing as much as is feasible about their own bodies and health. She could not, however, participate in a program that violated her religious beliefs. Her dilemma was whether to actively oppose the implementation of the program because of her uncertainty about which belief was of a higher order.

Part of Ms. Schwartz's ethical dilemma arises from what appears to be moral tension within the synagogue. While traditional orthodox Judaism is deeply committed to creation of new lives and is strongly opposed to abortion, another strand of thought in the Jewish community—more secularized and liberal—believes in the value of limiting fertility even through the practice of abortion. Particularly when the birth will be of an infant who is destined to a short, seriously debilitated life, abortion is an option that many people of Jewish origin take seriously.

Ms. Schwartz's congregation seems open enough to these practices that it wants to support a Tay Sachs screening program. Part of the problem may stem from the goal of discouraging engaged couples from procreating. This could come in the form of either discouraging marriage or discouraging childbearing within marriage. Neither is necessary to avoid giving birth to offspring afflicted with the disease provided one is willing to test and abort afflicted fetuses.

One argument sometimes given against this is that, with such an approach, two-thirds of the children born of parents who both are carriers will themselves be carriers. This would eventually increase the frequency of the gene in the population. Critics argue, however, that it will take a long time to significantly affect the gene pool and that the science of genetics is moving so rapidly that other technologies may be available to deal with that problem. Particularly if prenatal screening is available to identify fetuses with the actual disease, they believe that the slight increase in gene frequency is worth it if it would give couples a chance to bear children who are not afflicted with the disease.

There is some support for screening programs as a means of providing advance warning in order to give time for psychological, social, and medical preparation, even for couples who would continue with a pregnancy of an afflicted fetus. If that is a reason for the screening, then Ms. Schwartz might find reason to support it, even if she opposes abortion and discouraging of childbearing. Assuming Ms. Schwartz realizes that many couples will actually use the screening to limit fertility or to abort afflicted fetuses, is the possibility that some people will simply use the information for advance preparation a reason for Ms. Schwartz to support the program or is that merely a rationalization?

IN VITRO FERTILIZATION, SPERM DONATION, AND AID

Some of the most exotic and controversial developments in biomedical ethics involve our new-found capacity to manipulate the human egg and sperm cells in the laboratory in ways that permit the actual creation of human life in the "test tube."[10] These technologies were originally designed to help couples suffering from certain kinds of female infertility such as blockage of the oviduct to bypass the cause of the infertility. They involve removal of one or more egg cells from the ovary followed by fertilization mechanically in the clinic.

Some of the ethical problems have actually been with us for a long time. These newer technologies replicate what we have long been able to do through artificial insemination. They all raise the issues discussed earlier in this chapter of whether it is unethical to mechanically mimic the reproductive process. Some, especially within the Roman Catholic tradition, consider such manipulations "artificial," which is taken to mean "immoral."[11] Others see the moral issues not so much in the physical manipulation of the gametes per se, but in the risks of injury that are involved. Still others are concerned primarily about the more exotic uses of these technologies, which would permit conception of a child in ways that involve more than a married couple: first through artificial insemination by a donor and more recently through surrogate motherhood and schemes whereby a woman who wanted to bear a child that was genetically hers could engage another woman to carry the fetus through the pregnancy. The following two cases illustrate how allied health personnel will be involved in such issues, first, through artificial insemination and, second, through in vitro fertilization.

CASE 59: Fathering Through Sperm Donation: Can the Donor Know the Recipient?

A new department head in Obstetrics and Gynecology decides to expand the services offered by the department and acts to establish a fertility program. The program provides assessment, counseling, artificial insemination, and in vitro fertilization services. A laboratory is established to perform a range of services from sperm counts and frozen sperm storage to in vitro fertilization of ova from donors and natural mothers.

Frequently, the three technologists who work in the laboratory discussed the ethics and morality of the services offered by the fertility program. They felt pleased and personally rewarded that their work helped to make families happy. At the same time they felt uncertain about the morality of creating "unnatural" pregnancies. These discussions were theoretical and abstract as the activities did not affect their personal lives.

When artificial insemination was attempted with donor sperm, it was the responsibility of the laboratory to ensure an appropriate match. Blood type, tissue matching, biochemical profiling, family history as well as physical characteristics were considered in the selection of the sperm. An extensive data base was retained by the laboratory so that the match would produce a child who would appear to be the offspring of the husband as well as the mother.

When an attractive young black couple presented themselves to the fertility program because of their inability to conceive, it was learned that the husband's sperm count was very low and motility was reduced. Techniques for enhancing sperm count were attempted and failed. Attempts to fertilize one of the woman's ova with her husband's sperm, in vitro, also failed. They then requested artificial insemination with donor sperm.

Following a search of the records on all frozen sperm, the laboratory reported to the physician that no match was available. There were very few stored samples from black males, with none meeting the strict criteria that the program had established. Upon receiving this information the program director determined that it would be necessary to solicit a sperm donation from a likely male.

When discussing the procedure for solicitation with one technologist, the physician is interrupted by another technologist who enters the room. The conversation stops and the physician indicates that the technologist who just entered the room is just the person they are looking for. He is a black male of approximately the same skin coloring and body build as the client's husband, who comes from a professional family, is himself healthy, has children, and understands the procedures associated with artificial insemination.

The request to submit the necessary data collection and testing to ascertain his suitability as a sperm donor for this client presents the technologist with a true ethical dilemma. Because he has met the couple, he is uncertain of his ability to be objective about a child that might be conceived using his sperm. He must face and answer for himself the question of the fundamental morality of the process. He must determine his participation on the basis of his own ethical beliefs as well as his professional duty. What is the right thing to do?

The first question raised by this case is whether donor insemination is itself ethical. This raises not only questions about the artificiality of the conception process, but also significant issues about the involvement of a third party in the production of a baby.

Presumably both the woman and her husband would be informed that the sperm would be from a donor. (There are cases reported in which they are led to believe that the sperm is the husband's. This is sometimes done by mixing husband's and donor sperm. To the extent that the couple is not informed of the donor source, serious questions of veracity and fidelity to the commitments of the lay-professional relation are raised.)

If the technologist who has been approached is satisfied that the idea of donor insemination is, in principle, acceptable, he then must face the unique questions raised by this particular situation. He already knows the couple. Anonymity cannot be guaranteed. Of course, the couple could be kept ignorant of the source of the donation, but the technologist will know who has borne his child. He will even have access to their address and other identifying information. Presumably years later he could develop a desire to track down and communicate with "his" child.

Assuming that the couple is told of this risk, would it be ethically acceptable for the physician to make use of the available, ideal donor?

CASE 60: Making Babies in the Lab

The opportunity to participate in the improvement of the health of all persons was the driving rationale for John Morrow becoming a laboratory professional. He has enjoyed his various positions, feeling that his goal was achieved and that the work was rewarding. However, he now is uncomfortable about the role he is playing.

Three months ago Mr. Morrow accepted a transfer from the routine clinical laboratory of his hospital to a specialized in vitro fertilization clinic. His technical responsibilities include general chemistry and hematologic analyses of couples coming to the clinic, as well as the actual manipulation of the sperm and ova for in vitro fertilization. He is uncomfortable in his new role.

Mr. Morrow's discomfort arises from discussion with the clinic's clients, general news articles concerning difficulties associated with the use of this technology, and his own religious beliefs. Fundamentally, his concerns stem from an absence of ethical discussions among the clinic's staff. He does not believe that the clients are receiving adequate counseling nor have they given sufficient thought to questions of ethics.

Questions of creating then discarding life plague him. The "engineering" of children via the purposeful selection of specific sperm and the use of technology to overcome the vagaries of nature are dilemmas that demand more attention than he feels they are receiving.

Because his job is "technical" should he raise these questions?

Mr. Marrow's new position thrusts him into the middle of some of the most controversial and complex moral issues in health care today. Like the artificial insemination in Case 59, in vitro fertilization raises issues of whether it is unethical to manipulate the conception process and whether there is an "artificiality" about it that makes it unethical.

In vitro fertilization is more complex, however. Especially in the early days, there were serious questions of the risk to the offspring as well as to the woman. Now many of the basic safety issues appear to have been resolved, but other questions remain.

For technical reasons, it is standard to retrieve and fertilize several eggs at the same time, freezing extras for possible later implantation or cultivating several and selecting the most promising for implantation. The task of selecting and then discarding those not selected puts the health professional in a position that is awesome.

Frozen eggs raise another set of issues. They could be discarded once a conception has taken place, or they could be used elsewhere, either for research or for implantation into another woman, such as one who is infertile because of damaged ovaries.

One of the results of the professionalization of the allied health occupations is a questioning of the traditional view that roles such as Mr. Marrow's are merely "technical." If he is a laboratory professional, he will have a difficult time washing his hands of the moral issues raised by his work. Presumably, the physicians who run the clinic have answered these questions in their own minds, but that will not be sufficient. Mr. Marrow must decide whether he will take responsibility for the moral implications of the work he is doing in literally creating human life.

SURROGATE MOTHERHOOD

The very same technology that Mr. Marrow was using in Case 60 permits creation of life in the laboratory in ways that involve people who are not married couples. Once the egg is removed, it could be implanted into a woman who was not the source of the egg either to have her function as a surrogate, carrying the fetus to term for the purpose of returning it to the woman who supplied the egg, or to gestate a child she will not only give birth to but maintain after birth. In the latter case, the woman receiving the fertilized egg, the host mother, might be sterile due to damaged ovaries, but capable of maintaining a pregnancy. The egg could be fertilized by the host mother's husband's semen or she might be the recipient of extra fertilized eggs produced by another couple. Such arrangements add further complexity as is seen in the following case.

CASE 61: Parent by Proxy: Using a Cousin as a Surrogate Mother

Mr. and Mrs. Allen have seen Bernard Irwin, a physician assistant in a large fertility practice, for over five years for fertility studies and counseling. It has been determined that Mrs. Allen is infertile; both ovaries and uterus are damaged in ways that will not permit her to bear a child. After reviewing the various options available to them, the couple wishes to explore artificial insemination of a surrogate mother. Mrs. Allen's 35-year-old cousin has consented to serve as surrogate mother. She will be inseminated artificially with Mr. Allen's semen; the cousin will be the source of the egg for the conception.

The cousin is married and has four children of her own. A contract among the three has been developed and reviewed by an attorney.

During a follow-up office visit with Mr. Irwin, the couple and cousin present the plan to him and express their desire to proceed immediately. Mr. Irwin explains, "Although artificial insemination services are provided by the medical staff, this is an unusual request to artificially inseminate a wife's cousin with her husband's sperm." Questions were further raised about the cousin's husband's feelings. The cousin explains, "This is my body, and I want to do this for my family. What right do you have to ask these kinds of questions, after all, we've seen an attorney."

Being concerned about the rights of the cousin's husband and general feelings of discomfort, Mr. Irwin considered offering a referral to another provider in another state.

This case raises many complicated legal questions, such as whether the cousin's husband needs to be a party to the contract, whether the contract is legally binding should the cousin (or her husband) undergo a change of heart, and whether either Mr. or Mrs. Allen can legally become the parents of any child produced.

But Mr. Irwin also faces important moral issues if he is going to respond to the Allens' proposal. Surrogate motherhood raises all the issues of artificial insemination and in vitro fertilization seen in Cases 59 and 60. But it also raises serious questions about the relation of the host mother (and her husband) to the Allens. In this case, Mrs. Allen's cousin was also the source of the egg; she will be the genetic mother of the child. Whether she is the genetic mother or not, experience has shown that she may develop emotional bonds with the child she is gestating, raising questions about whether she should have the legal or moral right to change her mind. A liberal theory of ethics that emphasizes the rights and responsibilities of adults to make and keep agreements supports the view that if she contracts to turn the baby over to the Allens, she has a duty to do so. Critics argue, however, that the bonding between a pregnant woman and her fetus is something that is emotionally complex and cannot be understood in advance. They argue for the right to revoke the contract for a certain period after the birth. This raises the question, however, of whether such a stance, in effect, treats women as emotionally less than autonomous agents capable of making and keeping promises. The argument that supports the right to revoke the contract seems to claim that women are emotionally less than substantially autonomous agents.

Mr. Irwin must assess all these issues as well as his role in them. His proposed solution of a referral to another provider in another state could be designed to shift the case to a jurisdiction that has a more favorable set of surrogacy laws. But it also could be a way of trying to escape the moral judgments that need to be made. If he finds the procedures morally objectionable, is referral to another provider an adequate solution?

ENDNOTES

1. Richard T. Hull, *Ethical Issues in the New Reproductive Technologies* (Belmont, CA: Wadsworth, 1990).
2. John C. Fletcher, "The Morality and Ethics of Prenatal Diagnosis," in *Genetic Disorders and the Fetus*, ed. Aubrey Milunsky (New York: Plenum Press, 1979), pp. 621-635.
3. Daniel Bergsma, Marc Lappe, Richard O. Roblin, and James M. Gustafson, eds., *Ethical, Social and Legal Dimensions of Screening for Human Genetic Disease* (New York: Stratton Intercontinental Medical Book Corporation, 1974).
4. D. P. Wolf and M. M. Quigley, eds., *Human In Vitro Fertilization and Embryo Transfer* (New York: Plenum Press, 1984).
5. Larry Gostin, ed., *Surrogate Motherhood: Politics and Privacy* (Bloomington: Indiana University Press, 1990).
6. President's Commission for the Study of Ethical Problems in Medicine and Biomedical and Behavioral Research. *Splicing Life: The Social and Ethical Issues of Genetic Engineering with Human Beings* (Washington, DC: U.S. Government Printing Office, 1982); LeRoy Walters, "The Ethics of Human Gene Therapy," *Nature*, Vol. 320 (March 20, 1986), pp. 225-227.
7. President's Commission for the Study of Ethical Problems in Medicine and Biomedical and Behavioral Research, *Screening and Counseling for Genetic Conditions: The Ethical, Social, and Legal Implications of Genetic Screening, Counseling, and Education Programs* (Washington, DC: U.S. Government Printing Office, 1983).
8. Erving Goffman, *Stigma: Notes on the Management of Spoiled Identity* (Englewood Cliffs, NJ: Prentice Hall, 1963); Laurence B. McCullough, "The World Gained and the World Lost: Labeling the Mentally Retarded," *Ethics and Mental Retardation*, eds. Loretta Kopelman and John C. Moskop (Dordrecht, Holland: Reidel, 1984), pp. 99-118.
9. American Medical Association, Judicial Council, *Current Opinions of the Council on Ethical and Judicial Affairs of the American Medical Association: Including the Principles of Medical Ethics and Rules of the Council on Ethical and Judicial Affairs* (Chicago: AMA, 1989).
10. Paul Ramsey, *Fabricated Man* (New Haven, CT: Yale University Press, 1970).
11. Sacred Congregation for the Doctrine of the Faith, "Instruction on Respect for Human Life in Its Origin and on the Dignity of Procreation," *Origins*, Vol. 6, no. 40 (March 19, 1987), pp. 698-711.

CHAPTER 11

Mental Health and Behavior Control

Psychiatry and other forms of study and modification of human behavior raise many ethical problems in the allied health professions.[1] When we say that many people suffer from behavior disorders, we imply that they are harmed or injured by these conditions. To the extent that the health professions can assist in relieving that suffering or in modifying undesired behaviors, the traditional ethics of medicine that focuses on doing what will benefit the patient requires attempting to intervene. At the same time, we may lack consensus on whether the condition is really one requiring intervention. In the case of organically based illnesses, we can normally ask the patient or surrogate whether he or she wants help in attempting to change the condition. In the case of behavioral problems, however, there is often doubt whether the patient is capable of making an informed and rational choice. It is the consenting organ itself that may be "diseased." If we rely on surrogates, there may be significant conflicts of interest between the surrogate decision maker and the patient. The behavior of the patient may not bother the patient but can create inconvenience or embarrassment to the surrogate. Some of the most difficult ethical problems in the health care professions can arise in mental health and the behavioral sciences. In this chapter we look at cases raising these problems.

The first problem in dealing with mental health is with the concept of mental health itself. Traditionally, many mentally abnormal behaviors have been viewed as problems of religion or of criminality. Only in the last century have we begun to view these behaviors within the medical model. In the first section of this chapter we look at a case that raises the issue of the concept of mental health and whether mental problems should be deemed "deviant behavior choices" or "medical problems."

In the second section, we take up one of the classical ethical problems in the mental health professions—whether patients with mental health problems should be viewed as having sufficient autonomy that they can be asked to consent or refuse consent to treatment the way we would for organic medical treatments. The third section deals with the conflicts of interests that arise between the mental health patient and other parties—

other patients, families, work colleagues, or other members of the society. The problems here involve confidentiality, loyalty to the patient, and the trade-offs between patient interests and those of the others potentially affected by the patient's behavior.

Finally, in the fourth section of this chapter, we will focus on an example of other behavior controlling technologies—the use of electroshock on a mentally depressed patient.

THE CONCEPT OF MENTAL HEALTH

Human behavior is complex. It has been interpreted over the centuries in many different ways.[2] In traditional religious world views, members of the community who manifest strange behaviors might be thought to have been possessed by demons or to have been the victims of magical spells. We can say that the behavior is interpreted as religiously influenced deviance. The same behavior in another culture, also in a religious framework, might be interpreted as being sinful—as a violation of the will of God. While both are religious cultures, there is an important difference. While the view that sees the behavior as the result of demon possession or spells might imply that the behavior was not the "fault" of the individual (who could be called a "victim"), the behavior of the "sinner" is usually seen as somehow within the voluntary control of the actor.

In other cultures, the behavior may be seen as simply a "deviant life-style choice," not carrying any of the religious implications. Such behaviors may nevertheless be seen as socially unacceptable and in need of control. Especially if they harm others, they may be interpreted within a criminal model in which the behavior is illegal and worthy of social sanction.[3]

In still other interpretations the behavior is seen in what is called a "medical model." According to this now-dominant view, many unusual behaviors are believed to be caused by some medical condition. The convulsions we now associate with epilepsy are now thought to have an organic medical cause; they are not the result of demon possession, the wrath of God, or sinful life-style.

While we have fully medicalized some conditions that were once thought of in other terms, other behaviors are less clearly medical. Alcoholism, for instance, is believed by some to be a disease, while others continue to see it as a life-style choice or a sin. The medicalization of human behavior has very important and controversial implications. The choice of a "model" for interpretation of behavior does important work. It conveys an implied understanding of the source of the behavior, whether one is "responsible" for it, what experts or authorities should be consulted to deal with the behavior, and what interventions are to be used in attempting to modify the behavior.

The "medical model" in its pure form implies that there is an important "medical" (usually organic) element in the cause of the behavior.[4] It often implies that the individual manifesting the behavior is not volitionally responsible for it and is thus exempted from blame. It also implies that a medical professional is an appropriate expert for dealing with the behavior. Many of the most interesting and difficult ethical problems for those working in mental health arise at the point of classifying the patient's behavior as fitting in the medical model. The following case shows how allied health professionals may find themselves dealing with patients whose classification as medical is controversial.

CASE 62: Reality Orientation: Psychological Therapy or Social Oppression?

Joe Warriner, 27 years old, was admitted to a major county hospital where he was diagnosed with bacterial endocarditis and started on long-term antibiotic treatment. After a one-week stay in the county hospital, Mr. Warriner was transferred to a long-term care facility for prolonged antibiotic therapy, as he no longer had certifiable acute care needs for Medicaid reimbursement. The staff of the long-term facility anticipated a stay of at least five weeks to complete the medication regime. During the first 48 hours he became verbally abusive and threw a bed pan at a nurse on the night shift. A psychiatric consult was ordered by the attending physician. The psychiatrist took a history that revealed that Joe was a long-term street person with a history of intravenous drug abuse, antisocial behavior, and paranoid ideation. He wrote an order for Mr. Warriner to attend a "Reality Orientation and Socialization" group led by an occupational therapist and social worker.

In Mr. Warriner's first session of the group, he said that he had no need for the group, that he socialized just fine and understood the way things were on the street just fine. He proceeded to disrupt the group process, making negative comments to patients in the groups as well as the therapists. As the session came near to close, he said loudly, "This is a waste of my time, I'm just here to get medication for my heart and I don't want to talk to any of you social do-gooders or be in a group with all these psychos." Another patient took offense and started yelling at Mr. Warriner, and shortly the group escalated into a near showdown between him and two of the other members.

The therapists had to end the group session immediately and get Mr. Warriner back to his room. He continued to be agitated in the ward, and he insisted that he was not going back to the group.

The occupational therapist and the social worker were faced with the question of whether Mr. Warriner had a problem amenable to this therapy group or whether he had made a life-style choice that he didn't want to change at this point in time.

Mr. Warriner is what is often referred to as a difficult or "bad" patient. He is unpleasant to the point of being dangerous to other patients and staff. His antisocial behavior and paranoid ideation have at various points in history been interpreted as a bad attitude, possession by evil influences, or psychopathology. He could be seen as having made a life-style choice, as under religious influence, or as having a medical problem for which therapy was appropriate.

If he is seen as having a significant medical problem, there are important implications. He is less likely to be blamed for his behavior. He will be seen as a "patient" to be treated by a psychiatrist, occupational therapist, or social worker. The causal force that makes him behave strangely will be seen as organic or psychological rather than a voluntary choice or as resulting from some external source.

A person's behavior will be seen as "medical" if its cause is some organic lesion or chemical imbalance, especially if the lesion or imbalance was not the result of what is taken to be a voluntary choice on Mr. Warriner's part. If there is a brain lesion or a tumor causing abnormal hormonal secretions that cause him to behave in this peculiar way, it is unreasonable to blame him. Moreover, what he needs will be seen as within the medical realm: he needs a health care professional who has specialized knowledge capable of addressing his problems.

On the other hand, classifying his behavior within the medical model will be seen by some not only as mistaken, but offensive. If, for example, he is interpreted as rebelling against an immorally oppressive society, someone who labels him as having a "disease" will be seen as ignoring the real cause of his behavior—behavior that could be interpreted as morally appropriate rebellion. If he is interpreted as being punished by God or as having inherited bad karma from a previous life, then his behavior will be seen in an entirely different causal framework. He may be held accountable for his actions: either praised for rejecting societal oppression or blamed for his past deeds that condemned him to his present fate. Different kinds of expertise will be seen as appropriate: the clergy or the police perhaps. If he is seen as responding appropriately to an oppressive society, probably no professional expertise will be seen as needed at all. In fact, he could be viewed as a saint or martyr or hero. (Consider whether Gandhi, Malcolm X, Jesus, or Stalin could be classified as mentally ill by the psychiatrist who worked up Mr. Warriner.)

The issue raised by Mr. Warriner's case is what it takes for a person to be classified as a patient, as one in need of the services of health care professionals.

One condition seems to be that something bad is happening. Only if his behavior is interpreted as inappropriate and negative will he be seen as in need of health care services. But more than that will be needed. His behavior must be seen as having a significant organic (or psychological) component. If evil spirits, divine forces, or freely chosen life-style causes him to act the way he is acting, the behavior will be seen as less likely to fit the medical model. If there is believed to be a significant medical (organic-psychological) component causing his behavior, then it is more likely that those with the appropriate medical or psychological expertise will be seen as having something to offer. Finally, if the behavior is beyond his control (even if perhaps he was in some way originally responsible for the events that led to it), it is less likely he will be seen as blameworthy. For example, if his use of the intravenous drugs is seen as an "addiction" beyond personal control, then he presumably cannot be blamed for his present actions (although he might still be considered responsible for the choices that led him to start down the road to such use).

MENTAL ILLNESS AND AUTONOMOUS BEHAVIOR

Once we have reached agreement that the patient's condition is appropriately classified as a medical or health problem and therefore the appropriate concern of those in the mental health profession, the next issue to be confronted is whether the patient can nevertheless be sufficiently autonomous to consent or refuse consent for medical treatment.

As we discovered in Chapter 5, autonomy is both a psychological and a moral concept. One is said to be *psychologically* autonomous if one has substantial capacity to form a life plan and make choices in accord with it. Individual actions are autonomous to the extent that they are made in accord with such a life plan. Seen in this light, it becomes apparent that no person and no personal action can be said to be totally autonomous. Individual actions can be more or less autonomous depending on the degree to which the individual generates a decision based on his or her life plan.

Autonomy is also a *moral* concept. We saw in Chapter 5 that autonomy as a moral principle holds that actions are morally right to the extent that they respect the autonomous choices of individuals. We saw that informed consent as a moral requirement is grounded largely in the moral principle of autonomy.

In order for the moral principle of autonomy to come into play, however, the individual must be deemed to be a substantially autonomous agent. For many patients this decision is relatively easy. All minors are presumed not to have sufficient autonomy to make their own medical choices except in special circumstances. In special cases minors may be found to be mature and granted both the moral and legal right to consent to treatment on their own.[5] Some adults are so severely retarded or comatose that it is obvious they also are not significantly autonomous agents. On the other hand, most adults are sufficiently autonomous that they will clearly be treated as autonomous for purposes of making medical decisions. Even some people who are seeking mental health services are autonomous. The courts have determined that it is possible that a patient might be committed for mental treatment and still sufficiently autonomous that he or she is deemed mentally competent for purposes of consenting to or refusing treatment.[6] This is particularly true for certain critical medical treatments including electroshock.[7]

While autonomy is a moral and psychological category, competence is a legal category. Only a court can make a legal finding that a patient is incompetent to consent or refuse consent for treatment.

Nevertheless a significant number of patients receiving mental health services present serious problems at the borders of autonomy. For these cases autonomy must be viewed as a threshold concept.[8] A patient must be deemed either sufficiently autonomous that his or her own judgments will be accepted or below the threshold, in which case some surrogate will have to be designated for that purpose. The following two cases pose problems at the borderline of assessing autonomy in mental health treatment.

CASE 63: The Drug-Addicted Spinal Cord Patient: May He Refuse Treatment?

Jennifer Harwick is an occupational therapist in a large city hospital. She received a referral to see Dan Musto, a 23-year-old client. Mr. Musto had a spinal cord injury at the C-7 level that rendered him quadriplegic and had been discharged from the hospital after rehabilitation. Ms. Harwick's job as an occupational therapist was to provide a home evaluation and recommend environmental adaptations to make it possible for Mr. Musto to be more independent and safe in his home.

On her first home visit, while evaluating the bathroom in the house for safe tub transfers, she saw various pieces of what looked to her like drug paraphernalia. She left feeling somewhat uncomfortable, but decided to focus on the task at hand and did not ask him about the items.

When she arrived for her second home visit, she found Mr. Musto in the living room with two friends. It appeared to her that they were all high, and she noticed needles and syringes on the coffee table. She directly asked Mr. Musto if he was using drugs and he said "yes." He went on to say, "It's really none of your business what I do with my personal life, so don't bother trying to give me advice on quitting or getting help." Ms. Harwick told Mr. Musto that she was there to continue working on home adaptations and self-care skills, that it was time to start, and that he would need to ask his friends to leave for the hour. Mr. Musto became hostile and said, "They'll stay as long as I want them to, and anyway I'm not interested in therapy." Ms. Harwick attempted to talk with Mr. Musto about goals for therapy, but found him to be distracted and uncooperative, so she left. As she left the house, he yelled at her, "And don't bother coming back; I don't want your help."

She returned to the hospital at the end of the day to document the home health visits she had made and found herself pondering the dilemma of what to do about the incident in Mr. Musto's house. She reported to her supervisor that one of her cousins had almost died of a drug overdose and that she felt strongly about illegal drugs. She said she did not want to walk into a situation again where drugs were being used. Her supervisor told her that it was her obligation to provide the occupational therapy services for which Mr. Musto was referred and that his drug problem was not addressed in the doctor's referral. Further, if Mr. Musto was to continue living at home independently, he needed to learn proper transfer techniques to and from his bed and the tub and also to adapt his home for wheelchair safety. Without these interventions, he would need ongoing attendant care or placement in an extended care facility. What should Ms. Harwick do?

One of the firm conclusions of the moral debate about health care in the last half of the twentieth century is that competent patients have the moral and legal right to refuse any medical treatment provided that treatment is offered for the patient's own good. We saw in Chapter 5 that the moral principle of autonomy affirms the right of such patients to make their own choices even if they turn out to be bad decisions. In Chapter 13 we shall see that this right to refuse treatment is widely believed to hold even in cases in which the result of the refusal is likely to be death.

Mr. Musto is probably not making a life-and-death decision when he demands that Ms. Harwick stay away, although the consequences of the refusal are likely to be a much less mobile life for Mr. Musto. There may even be significant risk of injury and even a remote risk of death.

But Mr. Musto's right to refuse treatment is premised on the assumption that he is substantially mentally competent. It means nothing to hold out the moral principle of autonomy if the patient is not significantly an autonomous agent. How should Ms. Harwick go about assessing whether Mr. Musto is substantially autonomous?

Two elements might cause her concern. First, he is apparently a user of some injectable drug. Should the fact that he uses such drugs be sufficient for him to be deemed nonautonomous? Second, he has suffered a significant spinal cord injury that may well have left him depressed or otherwise injured psychologically. If Mr. Musto is not an autonomous agent, then if Ms. Harwick follows his demand not to be treated, she cannot be said to be respecting his autonomy. In fact, she may also be failing in the duties of beneficence. She will be failing to provide him with the benefits she is capable of bestowing. Should she treat Mr. Musto as an autonomous agent capable of refusing treatment, or should she take action on the basis that he may not be autonomous?

If she believes he may not be autonomous, what does she need to do to confirm that suspicion? Ms. Harwick is an occupational therapist. Does she have the capacity to determine whether he is living his life voluntarily according to a life plan that he has chosen? If not, who can help her? Psychiatrists cannot legally declare a patient to be incompetent; only a court can do that. Should she entertain a plan of going to court to get Mr. Musto declared incompetent? What other choices are available to her if she is not to honor his wishes? Is there any way that she can provide the training she thinks would benefit him if he is militantly refusing it?

The problem of assessing mental competency of psychiatric patients also arises in patients who are potentially suicidal. Some people argue that the very fact that one is suicidal is evidence that one is mentally incompetent. Others claim that some patients who are suicidal can have made rational, mentally competent, judgments that it is appropriate to end their lives. They hold that these people may have a clear understanding of their life options and that, all things considered, suicide is the best course. This might happen in the case of someone who has committed such a terrible wrong that he will never be able to escape the anguish. For example, a private pilot who was advised it was too dangerous to fly nevertheless took his entire family up, crashed the plane, and was the only survivor. After years of mental torment over what he had done, he ended his life believing there would never be any escape.

Another group who are sometimes claimed to commit suicide while rational are those with chronic, incurable, burdensome illness. The following case presents as example.

CASE 64: Is Suicide Ever the Rational Choice?

Diane Darlington, who is 46 years old, was admitted to an acute care psychiatric ward with suicidal ideation secondary to multiple medical problems including chronic diabetes, gastric ulcer, peripheral neuropathy, high blood pressure, retinopathy, and Raynaud's disease. Her symptoms included hypersomnia, decreased energy, decreased appetite with a loss of 100 pounds in the last year, decreased concentration, hopelessness, and anhedonia. Within the first 24 hours she was assessed by all team members including Sharon Spagnoli, the occupational therapist. In an occupational therapy group, Ms. Darlington participated minimally, until the topic of death came up. At this point she stated, "I'm tired of doing everything I'm supposed to do and not getting any better. I want to get totally well or die." She went on to talk about how hopeless her future was because her diabetes will lead both to physical and mental deterioration and leave her a vegetable. She says she is a member of the Hemlock Society and has decided to euthanize herself before she gets to that point. The group was taken aback, but tried to convince Ms. Darlington that she could work on her problems and still lead a satisfying life.

When Ms. Spagnoli reported this at the team meeting, there was a divided response. Some felt that Ms. Darlington should be assisted in alleviating her major depression, but if she should continue to choose to die, it was certainly her right. Ms. Spagnoli, the occupational therapist, felt strongly that Ms. Darlington needed therapy that would assist her in overcoming and facing her current and future disabling medical conditions. She suggested working with Ms. Darlington on nutritional issues, general health and fitness, as well as her self image. Ms. Spagnoli was very concerned that some team members appeared almost cavalier in their acceptance of Ms. Darlington's death wish. What should she do?

As in the previous case, one issue raised is whether Ms. Darlington is mentally competent to make her own decisions, even those that pose a serious risk to her life. Since Ms. Spagnoli is presumably not the one who should make a final decision about whether Ms. Darlington is mentally competent, she might urge other members of the health care team to undertake an initial assessment of competence. Should they attempt to have their patient restrained on grounds she is not competent? Should they make the attempt on grounds that she is of danger to herself (even if she is mentally capable of understanding what she is doing and therefore is substantially autonomous in her choice to take her own life)?

Assuming she is deemed to be autonomous enough to understand the nature of the choice she is making and is undertaking it in a substantially voluntary way, does Ms. Spagnoli or other members of the health care team have a moral or legal basis for intervening? The patient used the newly constructed term "euthanize" to refer to what she contemplates. There is a movement to legalize such active killing of terminally and critically ill patients. Some people claim that such euthanasia is morally and legally different from suicide, but others claim that the same moral arguments supporting the right to euthanasia while terminally or critically ill also support suicide in other conditions. Should Ms. Darlington's plan be considered euthanasia, suicide, or assisted suicide, and does it make any difference morally? For a further exploration of these issues see the cases in Chapters 8 and 14.

MENTAL ILLNESS AND THIRD-PARTY INTERESTS

The decisions in the previous section of this chapter posed traditional medical ethical questions of the conflict between benefiting the patient and protecting the patient's autonomy to the extent that it exists. Patients receiving mental health treatment also pose the newer ethical problems of conflict between the interests of the patient and the interests of others in the society. These can arise in the context of confidentiality. (See Chapter 7 for additional cases involving the general problem of breaking confidence in order to protect the interests of others.) Other conflicts between the interests of mental health patients and others include situations in which providing good care for the patient will necessarily jeopardize the care that can be given to others. Sometimes these problems arise because of the shortage of resources.

In the following case providing the beneficial therapeutic outing for one disturbed boy will create significant burdens for a therapist in a psychiatric facility. It also compromises the interests of other patients.

CASE 65: Sacrifice the One for the Good of the Many?

Jenny Markowitz, a therapist who worked in a psychiatric facility for children, shared the following practice dilemma.

"We had a boy here, Billy Thompson… who runs a lot. He was very dangerous to himself. Several times he got out of the building, and he could climb up on the ledge where there are steep, steep hills. He would go on the edge and threaten that he was going to jump. This past week we were going to take the kids to a lake. His teacher and I felt that it was totally ridiculous for this boy to be allowed to go on the trip. He would have to be kept on `hand-to-hand,' which means that he has to be on my hand at all times in order to control his running.

"I called the child's psychiatrist and explained how I felt. I also explained that I would not only have to staff this boy, but I would be responsible for other children as well. The week before we went on another trip I happened to be staffing the same child, and he was all over the place. It was not good for the other children I was staffing because they were totally ignored—I mean completely—and it really wasn't fair. This boy is very impulsive so you have to be right there all the time. Anyway, I explained my feelings to his psychiatrist, Dr. Morton Swazey, and told him that we had told the boy that we would not let him go any place where he might hurt himself.

"It really got to be a big issue because the psychiatrist thought the teacher and I were exaggerating. So we received a memo from the head supervisor telling us that we needed to consult with the psychiatrist. We did consult with him. An emergency meeting was called. It got to be ridiculous. As it ended up the team decided that the boy should go to the lake."

What should Ms. Markowitz do? Why?*

This case is reminiscent of those in Chapter 4 dealing with allocation of scarce resources. The therapist surely would claim that the problem would be solved if only the facility were provided adequate resources to give each child the supervision needed. That, however, is not likely to happen, at least in the short term. Ms. Markowitz will undoubtedly have to deal with her problem with the resources that are available.

**This case was submitted by Professor Ruth A. Hansen Ph.D., OTR.*

The central ethical issue is how to allocate Ms. Markowitz's scarce and valuable attention. She is in a situation where if she benefits one quite disturbed child needing her attention she will do so compromising the welfare of other children who may not be in as great a danger, but surely can benefit from the outing. Giving the hand-to-hand attention to Billy Thompson will result in the compromising of the interests of the other children.

Consider two ways of making the comparison among the claims of these children, ways that were explored in more detail in Chapter 4. First, Ms. Markowitz could try to estimate the benefits and harms to each child if she takes Billy on the outing to the lake. Billy clearly would benefit, but the other children would be exposed to some disadvantage. They would not get the attention of Ms. Markowitz and might even be at some risk of physical injury. Then Ms. Markowitz could try to estimate the benefits and harms to each child if she left Billy back at the facility so she could give more attention to the other children.

In this first approach, what is called the utilitarian approach, she would compare the sum of the envisioned net benefits (expected benefits minus expected harms) for each child from the two alternatives. The morally correct course would be the one that does the greatest net good for the group of children taken as a whole. If Billy were to gain more than the other children (taken as a whole) would lose by taking Billy along, then Ms. Markowitz should take him. But if she concluded that the total loss to the other children if Billy were taken on the trip exceeded the gain to Billy, then morally she ought to leave him behind. That is the way a utilitarian would sort out the competing claims.

Using this first approach, however, omits a question that Ms. Markowitz may have been asking. It omits any consideration of fairness or justice. Fairness or justice focuses not only on the total amount of good that is done, but also on how the good is distributed. According to the principle of justice, each child should get his or her "due." Depending on one's interpretation of the principle of justice, that could mean that each person should have an equal chance of the benefit of the lake outing. Perhaps Ms. Markowitz would take Billy one time and the other children as a group another time, giving each child one chance at an outing. Of course, under that plan the other children would get half the outing experience they would otherwise get.

Some egalitarian interpretations of the principle of justice provide a different emphasis. Holders of this view would point out that not all the children are equally needy. One egalitarian interpretation of justice holds that the fair arrangement is to give the benefits to the most needy or worst off patient (even though the total amount of good might be less than other alternative arrangements). Can we tell from the case whether Billy is worse off than the other children?

Assuming he were the worst off, an egalitarian who focuses on need would claim that Ms. Markowitz should give special attention to Billy even if the total good she did (summing the expected benefits and harms for all the children affected) were less than if she left him out. Do you think Billy has a special claim of justice to Ms. Markowitz's attention?

Finally, consider the perspective of the psychiatrist in this case. Assume that Dr. Swazey is committed morally to the traditional Hippocratic view that his moral duty is to do what is in the best interest of his patient. Assuming he really believes that the outing would be good for Billy (better than staying behind in the facility), he would apparently have to insist that from his point of view Billy should go on the outing. If this is so, what purpose is served when Ms. Markowitz telephones Dr. Swazey? He would have a moral duty to ignore the interests of those who are not his patients and support Billy's participation provided that he believed it would be better for him than leaving him behind. Should she be bound by his opinion or is she in a different moral position, one in which she must balance the competing claims of different children? What role should the physician responsible for the welfare of the individual patient have in deciding how to allocate scarce resources among the patients in the psychiatric facility?

The conflict of interest between psychiatric patients and others may extend well beyond the competition for a therapist's attention. In the following case an occupational therapist must deal with such a conflict in dealing with an HIV-positive patient whose behaviors pose risks to others—not only other patients, but staff, students, and visitors as well.

CASE 66: A Manic Patient Who Is HIV+ — The Welfare of Others

Michael Perry is an occupational therapist working in a state psychiatric hospital. One patient in his unit is diagnosed with bipolar disorder and AIDS-related complex (ARC). This patient has a long history of bipolar disorder. In recent manic episodes she has shown increased aggression toward other patients and staff. This patient is considered to be an escape risk. Currently she is in a hypermanic phase characterized by hypersexism, poor insight, and lack of control. She has been smearing blood and other body fluids and is threatening to smear them on patients and staff. Three concerns that the staff has are:

1. What are this patient's rights—especially related to confidentiality, seclusion, and use of restraints?
2. What are the rights of other patients, visitors, and staff?
3. How much information should be shared with students who are on the unit four hours each week?

In Chapter 7 we examined the ethical principle of fidelity and its implication for the promise of confidentiality. We found that there is in health professional ethics a general implied promise of confidentiality. Two major exceptions that would plausibly limit such a promise, however, involve cases in which keeping a confidence would pose a significant threat of harm to the patient and those in which keeping the confidence would pose a significant threat of harm to others.

Breaking confidence solely to benefit the patient was traditionally justified in older paternalistic ethics of the Hippocratic form. We saw that in some codes of allied health professionals the paternalistic exception is still included. For example, some codes, such as the physician assistant's, retain the authorization to break confidence for the benefit of the patient, but add provisions authorizing breaking confidence for the benefit of others in the community.[9] Increasingly, the paternalistic reason for breaking confidence is being dropped altogether. For example, the American Society for Medical Technology[10] and the American Occupational Therapy Association[11] codes do not include such an exception. The emergence of the principle of autonomy has come to be seen as overriding any paternalistic reasons for breaking confidence.

Is there any reason why Michael Perry would be inclined to break confidence to benefit the patient in this case? If so, should she be viewed as an autonomous patient who has the right to have confidences kept, or does the fact that she is institutionalized in a state psychiatric facility prove that she is not sufficiently autonomous to make such judgments? If she is not mentally competent, then presumably a guardian is responsible for making medical judgments including consenting to medical treatment. At the least, this guardian would have to know about the patient's medical condition in order to make informed choices. Could the guardian waive the patient's right to consent the way a competent patient could?

The other major reason why confidences might be broken does not rely on paternalistic reasoning focusing on benefit to the patient. It focuses on the interests of others. While some codes have held that any benefit to others in society would justify breaking confidences, most today, if they include an exception to the confidentiality rule in order to benefit other parties, insist that the benefit be very carefully defined. For example, the American Medical Association endorses breaking confidence to permit the physician to take "reasonable precautions" to protect the intended victim (including notification of law enforcement authorities) if "a patient threatens to inflict serious bodily harm to another person and there is a reasonable probability that the patient may carry out the threat."[12]

That provision originally was applied to psychiatric patients who threatened to assault or even kill others.[13] The reasoning would seem to apply, at least in principle, to patients who threaten to infect others with HIV-infected body fluids. In this case there is certainly a reasonable probability that the patient will carry out the threat; she, in fact, is already smearing blood and other body fluids.

The real question is whether the risk to others if they contact the patient's blood poses a significant threat of "serious bodily harm." Contacting the blood is not the same as murder, but it surely is not to be taken lightly. Does the reasoning that would permit violating the patient's confidence when there is a serious threat to others apply in this case?

If so, is there any morally significant difference between warning staff, other patients, visitors, or students? On the one hand, staff routinely handle confidential patient information. They should have the insight and discipline necessary to maintain the confidence. But they get information on a "need-to-know" basis. Traditionally, the need to know was presumed to be based on the interests of the patient, not the interests of the staff. Moreover, the staff ought to be schooled in universal precautions to protect against infected blood products so that their risk could actually be considered smaller than that to patients, visitors, and students.

Presumably the patients are also mentally incapacitated, which might make it more difficult to presume that they can protect themselves against such risks and, in any case, would raise questions about their ability to consent to risk of exposures. Is there any moral basis for treating these groups of people who are at risk any differently when it comes to deciding whether to inform them of the risk this patient poses?

OTHER BEHAVIOR-CONTROLLING THERAPIES

The ethical problems of mental health arise not only in clinical psychology; they must be faced in other behavior-controlling interventions as well. Neurological interventions including psychosurgery and electroshock require judgments about the concept of mental health. They require judgments about when a patient is autonomous; they require moral trade-offs between the welfare of the patient and that of other parties.

Electroshock involves administering electrical charges at voltages high enough to cause convulsions. In some forms, if muscle relaxant medication is not administered, the force has been known to be strong enough to cause breakage of bones. The exact effect on the brain is not known, but some patients are reportedly improved as a result of the shock.

This imagery of convulsions and brute physical assault raises doubts in some people's minds about the acceptability of electroshock therapy (ECT). Especially, as in the following case in which the patient appears to have changed her mind, the allied health worker involved in electroshock faces serious moral issues.

CASE 67: Withdrawing Consent for Electroshock

Janet Westwood, a severely depressed widow of 58, was being treated with antidepressant medications. After being given fair trials of two medications, she was not experiencing sufficient relief from her depression. She still was refusing to eat and continued to display suicidal ideation. The team discussed the case at length, and the psychiatrist (Milton Williams), the nurse (Donna Thompson), and social worker (Sylvia Rathman) all agreed that electroshock therapy should be tried. Ann Benson, the occupational therapist, disagreed. She said that she had seen some small gains in therapy groups relative to attention span and motivation. Ms. Benson thought that more time should be given to evaluate the effect of medications. But the consensus of the group was to proceed with electroshock therapy.

The patient, Mrs. Westwood, was asked to sign consent papers to receive electroshock treatment. The nursing staff told her that the team had agreed that this would be the best thing for her.

During her six-week hospitalization, Mrs. Westwood had come to trust and talk openly to Ms. Benson. After one of the occupational therapy groups, Mrs. Westwood pulled Ms. Benson aside and told her that she needed to talk with her confidentially about something and pleaded with Ms. Benson to listen to her. Mrs. Westwood told Ms. Benson that she did not want electroshock therapy and that she thought the doctor was treating her this way because he didn't care about older people and just wanted her out of his hair. She said to Ms. Benson, "Really, I am feeling much better and I don't want these treatments. Do you think that I need them?"

Ms. Benson felt torn about what to say. She saw Mrs. Westwood's point about how older women with depression are sometimes treated and had herself questioned the advisability of ECT without giving more time for the antidepressant medications to work.

Should Ms. Benson tell Mrs. Westwood that the electroshock treatment is a good idea and what Mrs. Westwood needs, and thus support the doctor and the team? Or should she tell Mrs. Westwood what she really thinks: that the electroshock treatment is premature, that the medicine should be tried for a longer time period, and that she does not think that Mrs. Westwood needs the treatment at this time? Should Ms. Benson tell Mrs. Westwood about the discussions of the medical team and her own statements at the meeting?

Traditional health care ethics would view this case as one in which the physician has made a clinical judgment that he believes electroshock is best for Mrs. Westwood. The views of the occupational therapist, the nurse, and the social worker would not be important. But newer approaches to ethics raise the question of consent and the role of the patient in choosing between the electroshock and medication.

Deciding that depression is a medical condition in need of therapy is, in itself, a matter that some would consider questionable. It raises the question in earlier cases in this chapter of what counts as a health matter. But assuming that therapies have a plausible chance of changing the course of Mrs. Westwood's depression, Ms. Benson will have to decide whether the traditional physician authority of the Hippocratic model should prevail or whether the patient's own view should be controlling. The issues of informed consent will be addressed more fully in the cases of Chapter 13, but they must be confronted here.

Before she can invoke the notions of informed consent, a judgment will have to be made about whether Mrs. Westwood retains autonomy to make any judgments about her care in her present condition. Is there reason to believe Mrs. Westwood is capable of deciding about electroshock in her depressed state? If she lacks competence, what is the significance of her psychiatrist asking her to consent to the electroshock in the first place? If she is capable of consenting to the electroshock, is she also capable of withdrawing that consent?

Regardless of whether Mrs. Westwood is considered sufficiently autonomous to consent or refuse consent to electroshock, both she and Ms. Benson must compare the risks and benefits of electroshock and pharmacological antidepressants. Ms. Benson seems to think that electroshock should be resisted. Since it has a record of successful treatment of depression and the drug therapy has not proved effective for Mrs. Westwood, what would lead them to resist the electroshock? Is it that one is electrical and the other chemical, that one is so dramatic compared to the other, or that one is more poorly understood? We often think of drug therapies as temporary and reversible while other behavior-controlling therapies are more permanent. Is it a virtue or a flaw of a therapy that it has a more permanent effect? Ms. Benson seems concerned both about Mrs. Westwood's views and about her own sense of doubt about ECT. Which should guide her in deciding what to say about the treatment?

ENDNOTES

1. Sidney Bloch and Paul Chodoff, eds., *Psychiatric Ethics* (New York: Oxford University Press, 1981); Max Rosenbaum, ed., *Ethics and Values in Psychotherapy: A Guidebook* (New York: The Free Press, 1982); H. Tristram Engelhardt and Laurence B. McCullough, "Ethics in Psychiatry," in *American Handbook of Psychiatry*, 2nd ed., Vol. 7 (New York: Basic Books, 1981), pp. 795-818; American Psychiatric Association, *Ethics Committee Opinions of the Ethics Committee on the Principles of Medical Ethics with Annotations Especially Applicable to Psychiatry*, 1989 Edition (Washington, DC: APA, 1989); Amnon Carmi, Stanley Schneider, and Albert Hefez, *Psychiatry—Law and Ethics* (New York: Springer-Verlag, 1986); David K. Kentsmith, Susan A. Salladay, and Pamela A. Miya, *Ethics in Mental Health Practice* (New York: Grune and Stratton, 1986); Loretta Kopelman and John C. Moskop, *Ethics and Mental Retardation* (Boston: D. Reidel, 1984); and Ruth Macklin, *Man, Mind, and Morality: The Ethics of Behavior Control* (Englewood Cliffs, NJ: Prentice Hall, 1982).
2. Arthur L. Caplan, H. Tristram Engelhardt, and James J. McCartney, *Concepts of Health and Disease: Interdisciplinary Perspectives* (Reading, MA: Addison-Wesley, 1981).
3. Antony Flew, "Disease and Mental Illness," *Crime or Disease?* (London: Macmillan, 1973), pp. 38-48.
4. Robert M. Veatch, "The Medical Model: Its Nature and Problems," *Hastings Center Studies*, Vol. 1, no. 3 (1973), pp. 59-76. Also see Talcott Parsons, *The Social System*, Chap. 9 (New York: The Free Press, 1951).
5. Joseph Goldstein, "Medical Care for the Child at Risk: On State Supervention of Parental Authority," *Yale Law Journal*, Vol. 86 (1977), pp. 669-670.
6. *In re Maida Yetter*, 62 Pa.D. and C.2d 619 (1973).
7. *New York City Health and Hospitals Corporation* v. *Stein*. 335 N.Y.S.2d 461 (1972).
8. Ruth Faden and Tom L. Beauchamp in collaboration with Nancy N. P. King, *A History and Theory of Informed Consent* (New York: Oxford University Press, 1986), pp. 235-269.
9. American Academy of Physician Assistants, *Code of Ethics of the Physician Assistant Profession* (Alexandria, VA: AAPA, adopted 1983, amended 1985 House of Delegates).

10. American Society for Medical Technology, *Code of Ethics* (Washington, DC: ASMT, n.d.).
11. American Occupational Therapy Association, *Occupational Therapy Code of Ethics*, 1994.
12. American Medical Association, *Current Opinions of the Council on Ethical and Judicial Affairs of the American Medical Association: Including the Principles of Medical Ethics and Rules of the Council on Ethical and Judicial Affairs* (Chicago: AMA, 1989), p. 21.
13. *Tarasoff* v. *Regents of University of California.* 17C.3d 425, 131 Cal. Rptr. 14, 551 P.2d 334, in Thomas A. Shannon and Jo Ann Manfra, eds., *Law and Bioethics: Texts with Commentary on Major U.S. Court Decisions* (New York: Paulist Press, 1982), pp. 293-319.

CHAPTER 12

Experimentation on Human Subjects

Many of the great controversies in health care ethics have focused on problems in research involving human subjects. The research done by the Nazis gave rise to the Nuremberg trials that exposed to all humankind the outrageous things that could be done in the name of medical science. Those trials gave rise to the Nuremberg Code, 1946,[1] the first publicly written international document setting out an ethic for research on human subjects.

It may come as a surprise to some that, taken literally, the Hippocratic ethic does not permit research on human subjects, at least if it is designed to gain knowledge rather than to help a specific patient. The code says that everything a health care worker does should be to benefit the patient according to the clinician's ability and judgment. It is the very nature of medical research that the purpose is not to benefit the individual subject, but to produce generalizable knowledge for the benefit of the future of the people as a whole. The various codes of ethics of the allied health professions vary considerably on these matters. Some follow the Hippocratic Oath in pledging commitment to the welfare of the individual patient. The American Physical Therapy Association, for instance, says that "Physical therapists are to be guided at all times by concern for the physical, psychological, and socioeconomic welfare of those individuals entrusted to their care."[2] That does not include doing things to patients for the purpose of producing generalizable knowledge. Others just as clearly expand the health care provider's responsibility to include the interests of society. The American Dietetic Association, for instance, proclaims in its code that the practitioner has an obligation to society as well as the client.[3] The American Academy of Physician Assistants says that the physician assistant should be committed to the "health, safety, welfare, and dignity of all humans," which would seem to justify involvement in research, not just individual patient care.[4] The American Speech-Language-Hearing Association specifically acknowledges that its members participate in research.[5]

Health professionals have, of course, faced difficult situations in which known therapies were not successful. In some of these cases, they might, in desperation, try something new, hoping it would help. Sometimes that might be called "experimenting," but it is not medical research as we now know it. Trying something new on a patient is what can be called "innovative therapy." It is used precisely as with any other therapy because it is believed, everything considered, to be the best thing to do for the patient.

Medical research in a more formal sense is quite different. It often involves randomization between two or more therapies. The therapies are chosen precisely because it is not known which is better. The process of randomization and many of the tests performed on the subjects are not done to benefit the patient; they are done to produce knowledge for society. Some of these experiments on human subjects may even involve normal subjects or patients who are not suffering from the condition being studied. They surely are not involved for their personal benefit. None of these research interventions could be justified in advance as being best for the individuals; none could be justified under the traditional Hippocratic ethic or any allied health profession code that holds its members to working solely for the welfare of the individual patient.

During the Nuremberg trials, a critical choice had to be made. Either the medical community could return to the Hippocratic notion that every intervention had to be for the benefit of the patient (thus eliminating randomized trials, systematic data gathering, and the use of normal subjects), or it could modify the Hippocratic tradition, providing exceptions in the case of medical research that would justify some actions by health professionals not based on the good of the immediate patient.

The health care community—and the world public—took the latter course. It developed an ethic that permitted "use" of human beings under certain carefully defined conditions. The Nuremberg Code spells out one version of these conditions. For one, the good being sought must be important and not obtainable by other means.[6] This requirement necessitates calculating the risks and benefits of the research proposal, a set of issues we shall take up in section one of this chapter. That would provide some protection, but not nearly enough. Theoretically, the Nazi experiments could have been designed to produce really important information not obtainable by other means.

To provide further protection, the writers of the Nuremberg Code placed as the first and perhaps most important new requirement, the provision that the consent of the subject be obtained. The code called voluntary consent "absolutely essential."[7] This, as we saw in Chapter 5, is grounded in the ethical principle of autonomy. Informed consent in research will be taken up in the last section of this chapter preparing the way for additional cases raising consent issues that will be covered in Chapter 13.

Other provisions in the Nuremberg Code include protection of privacy and confidentiality (to be explored in the second section of this chapter) and equity in subject selection (to be taken up in the third section).

In examining the ethics of research on human subjects, other professional and public codes that have emerged since the events of Nuremberg will be important to consider. The World Medical Association developed its Helsinki Declaration in 1964.[8] While covering many of the same requirements of Nuremberg, it is a professionally generated code—written by the world association of medical societies. In some ways it differs from Nuremberg, not only in its origins, but in its content as well. For example, while Nuremberg insists on the autonomous informed consent of all subjects, the Declaration of Helsinki recognizes that in some cases it is necessary to do research on infants, children, the severely retarded, or critically ill, who are not mentally capable of consenting. The notion of surrogate or guardian consent, and the moral limits of such consent, are introduced in the Helsinki Declaration.[9]

In the United States the American Medical Association adopted a specific code for research on human subjects in 1966.[10] The various professional associations of the allied health professions have spoken to varying degrees about involvement of their members in research with human subjects. Some, such as the occupational therapist's code, make brief mention of research on human subjects.[11] Some others, such as the American Speech-Language-Hearing Association, go into substantial detail.[12] Still others appear to assume that the allied health professional will not be directly involved in research with human subjects in a morally significant way.

In the public arena, the federal government of the United States began being concerned about protection of human subjects in the 1960s. By 1970 the first federal guidelines designed to protect human subjects were issued by the Department of Health, Education, and Welfare (DHEW, now called the Department of Health and Human Services, or DHHS).[13] With several dramatic cases involving alleged abuse of human subjects in the 1970s and 1980s, more formal regulations emerged including requirements that all research funded by the Department of Health and Human Services be reviewed by local institutional review boards (IRBs) made up of health professionals and laypeople capable of assuring that the welfare and rights of human subjects were adequately protected.[14] These were revised and extended to cover virtually all federal government research in 1991.[15] The following cases reveal some of the major problems raised in assessing the ethics of such research.

CALCULATING RISKS AND BENEFITS

The earliest efforts to protect human subjects focused on assessment of risks and benefits. As was fitting the earlier, more Hippocratic ethic focusing on benefiting patients and protecting them from harm, the primary attention of those reviewing research was directed to research posing significant risks. They were not as concerned about protecting the rights of subjects who were involved in research with little or no risk. They, for example, were not focused on the possible inequity of a research project conducted exclusively on low-income patients as long as they were not at substantial risk. They were not concerned about whether potential subjects gave their informed consent to be studied as long as they were not going to be placed at much risk of injury. By way of contrast, the allied health professions whose codes focus on research at all pay attention to at least some of these issues of rights of subjects as well as simply making sure the subjects are not injured. The American Speech-Language-Hearing Association, for instance, has not only included an explicit reference in its code to the necessity of getting subject consent,[16] they have, since 1982, promulgated a separate statement devoted entirely to ethics in research, which specifies many concerns beyond mere protection of subjects from risk. These include matters of honesty as well as confidentiality, plagiarism, and fraud.[17]

The older, more traditional, codes are much more limited, focusing only on benefits and harms to subjects. Assessing the benefits and harms and determining how the risks to the subjects should be related to the benefits envisioned for the society was the central task in the early years. The following case reveals some of the problems in making such assessments.

CASE 68: Risks in an Occupational Health Study

Marcy Mencovitz, as chief of the Occupational Therapy Department at the state's most prestigious research hospital, has served on its institutional review board for the past three years. The IRB is responsible for reviewing all research involving human subjects to assure that the subjects' rights and welfare are protected.

Having reviewed the 13 protocols for this month's meeting, she was not expecting much controversy over the one entitled "Assessment of Carcinogenic and Mutagenic Potential of Employment in the Organic Solvent Chemical Industry." As an occupational therapist, she had worked with patients who had suffered from chemical exposures and burns while working in the county's large chemical plants. She realizes the study is important.

She believes that the risks to the subjects are quite modest. Using the legal authority of the state's laws permitting occupational health assessments, the investigators are proposing to do a thorough record review of the plant's medical facility. They would also access from the payroll department records of time missed from work over the past 20 years. This would be combined with intensive interviews with present and former employees. A subsample would also be recruited for in-hospital exercise tolerance tests and a battery of other tests related to lung function. These would include administration of very modest doses of some of the chemicals these workers were exposed to in the plant. They would be administered through ventilators. Blood and urine samples would be studied for metabolites. Exposures were calculated to be equal to the typical ambient air levels in the plant.

The protocol claimed that none of these would be particularly stressful or dangerous and that workers would be compensated at their usual pay rates for time missed from work.

When the meeting begins, the lead reviewer presents a summary of the protocol. He seems to agree with Ms. Mencovitz that the risks are minimal. He recommends routine approval.

Then the other members of the committee are given an opportunity to question the protocol. Dr. Lenore Huntington, chief of the oncology research center at the hospital, waits until others have asked minor, routine questions. She begins probing the assessment of benefits and risks. She says she is concerned about the lung function and exercise tolerance tests on these workers. Many of them are in their fifties and sixties. Was there any evidence about the risks, say, of myocardial infarction, from workers who were not used to exercise?

Assured by the cardiologist on the committee that these risks were really quite modest, she then pursues the question of purposeful exposure of workers to potentially carcinogenic chemicals.

Several defenders of the protocol point out that since the workers are being taken off the job for the tests and the exposure levels are calculated to equal the exposure in the plant, there is no change in risk to the workers. In fact, since they would be exposed only briefly during the battery of tests, their day's exposure would actually be less than if they had been in the plant that day.

Dr. Huntington is not satisfied. She is not convinced that purposeful exposure of the subjects by the investigators to a potential carcinogen, even at low doses, is morally the same as exposures obtained by the workers through their daily work. She argues that even if the exposure levels are the same or lower, the experimental administration is unacceptable.

Then she introduces her real concern. She had often been the recipient of the IRB's aggressive questioning of the risks to which subjects were exposed in her oncology protocols. That questioning was often led by Dr. Ralph Goldstein, from the Department of Social Medicine, who is a co-investigator in this project. (Dr. Goldstein has excused himself from the meeting because of his conflict of interest in the chemical exposure protocol.)

Dr. Huntington says she thinks this is one of the most dangerous protocols she has seen come before the IRB. She says she is particularly concerned about the social and psychological risks of these workers. What would happen to them, she asks, if the blood levels are found to be unacceptably high or if former workers are found to have unusually high rates of cancer? Wouldn't the plant managers be forced to lay the high-risk workers off? Perhaps the plant would even be forced to close, costing these workers their jobs. These are workers who had been in these plants for many years and at their ages would be unlikely to find new work. She says she can envision whole industries being shut down, even the county employment base eroded. She claims that the risks are very significant. She urges a vote against the protocol as posing risks to the subjects and others that were beyond what is tolerable.

Ms. Mencovitz is stunned. What she had perceived to be a routine, low-risk protocol was being denounced by Dr. Huntington as one of the most dangerous protocols the IRB had ever seen. How should she assess the risks and benefits? How should she vote?

What is one person's simple, routine, valuable protocol is another's outrageously dangerous experimental intervention. Part of the problem here is perhaps an underlying feud between Drs. Huntington and Goldstein. Dr. Huntington perhaps sees this as the golden opportunity to ridicule Dr. Goldstein's persistent nagging criticisms of her oncology protocols. Dr. Huntington correctly believes that her oncology protocols are carefully planned and that harms to subjects (other than from their underlying disease) are quite modest. But is she taking her frustrations out on

Dr. Goldstein, and, if so, should that make any difference to Ms. Mencovitz if she believes Dr. Huntington has raised valid concerns?

The risks that Dr. Huntington has identified include both physical risks and social-psychological ones. The main physical risk is the exposure to the challenge doses of the plant chemicals. Should Ms. Mencovitz conclude that the risks are smaller than the normal plant exposures and therefore can be ignored, or does the fact that the potentially toxic substance is administered as part of the protocol make a difference?

The most difficult problem for Ms. Mencovitz is how she should assess the long-term risks that these subjects or their fellow workers who might lose their jobs if the plant is shut down because it is too dangerous. On the one hand, the entire purpose of the study is to identify such risks and help prevent exposures that are too dangerous. On the other hand, these workers may be worse off unemployed than if they continue their exposure to the chemicals. Since the plant has operated in the community for over 20 years and similar plants have existed much longer, the risk levels must be fairly modest, or the danger would have been recognized earlier. But it is precisely because there is concern about the risk level that the study is being undertaken. Should the risks to workers be explained to them so that they can refuse to participate in the study should they prefer to keep their jobs secure? Can they keep their jobs secure by individually refusing to participate if enough of their co-workers agree to be in the study so that the plant might not be shut down?

Finally, Ms. Mencovitz must consider Dr. Huntington's concern over the long-term effects on the town if the chemical industry is forced out. These may be the most serious risks of the study, yet they are surely the hardest to assess. Moreover, the current federal regulations governing IRBs specifically state that "The IRB should not consider possible long-range effects of applying knowledge gained in the research (for example, the possible effects of the research on public policy) as among those research risks that fall within the purview of its responsibility."[18] That seems to preclude the long-range concerns that Dr. Huntington was raising, but why should the IRB be mandated to exclude long-range public policy harms? It clearly considers potential long-range benefits of research, including potential benefits reflected in public policy. Why should Ms. Mencovitz be obliged to consider the long-range benefits but exclude the long-range harms?

PRIVACY AND CONFIDENTIALITY

A second major issue in the ethics of research involving human subjects is protection of privacy and confidentiality. The general issues of confidentiality were examined in Chapter 7. There we saw that one moral basis for the requirement that medical professionals maintain confidentiality is an implied promise to do so. If that is the basis, then the underlying moral principle is fidelity or promise-keeping. The key is then what is promised.

Traditional Hippocratic ethics would permit breaking of confidences when the clinician believed doing so would benefit the patient. Sometimes, of course, the patient might not agree with that judgment.

Newer codes, those reflecting a more patients' right approach, include a stronger confidentiality requirement. According to those, if the clinician believes that the patient could be benefited by disclosure of confidential medical information, he or she must ask the patient. If the patient agrees, there is no problem, but if the patient insists that the confidence be kept, then it must be.

The second basis for breaking confidence involves situations in which the clinician believes that disclosure will benefit not the patient, but others in society. That disclosure may be to other specific individuals or to law enforcement authorities. Many codes now accept the need to break confidence if there is a serious threat of bodily harm to others.

Confidentiality becomes a critical issue in research involving human subjects when medical information in a patient's chart could be useful in the research enterprise. Sometimes the risk is that others will be able to identify the patient as a subject of a study. In other cases, the problem is that the investigators themselves will obtain information that the patient does not want disclosed to strangers—even if they happen to be legitimate researchers.

Some researchers assume that it is acceptable to search a patient's medical records for research purposes provided that the patient is not identifiable in the published study. Others hold that even if the patient is not identifiable, the fact that investigators are entering the medical record itself constitutes a breach of confidentiality unless the patient has given permission. The following case reveals how confidentiality can arise in the research setting.

CASE 69: Protecting Privacy in Medical Research

In late September, with her 7-year-old finally settled into second grade with his permanent teacher after two weeks of substitutes and her 4-year-old daughter in nursery school, Susan Arnold, RRA, decided to accept an offer of part-time employment. The position, at an area teaching hospital, involved abstracting clinical data from patient medical records for an externally funded research study of Hashimoto's thyroiditis. Since there was no risk to the patients from the use of their data and the data would be collected in aggregate form without patient identifiers, the investigator believed that it qualified for an exemption from the review of the local institutional review board and that consent for the record search was not necessary.

While reviewing the record of a recently discharged patient for demographic data, she recognized the patient's name as that of her son's second grade teacher. On review of the record, she noted that although the first admission in the patient's record resulted in the diagnosis of Hashimoto's thyroiditis, the second and more recent admission indicated an admitting diagnosis of dysphagia and a final diagnosis of esophageal candidiasis. On further review of the record, she was dismayed to learn that her son's teacher, a 31-year-old man, had just been diagnosed with AIDS. Should Ms. Arnold have been allowed to conduct the record search without the patient's explicit consent? Would doing so violate the patient's right to confidentiality?

Current federal regulations permit certain exemptions to the general requirement that research involving human subjects must be reviewed and approved by a local institutional review board. These exemptions include studies in which there is no possibility of harm to the subject (such as record searches and the use of pathological and diagnostic specimens) provided their data are collected in such as way that there are no identifiers.[19] Some IRBs, however, have realized that there are rare cases in which subjects may object to the research even though they are not at risk. For example, some subjects may object to the purpose of some studies. Even though they cannot be hurt physically by the use of their records, they may nevertheless be offended—and have their autonomy violated—if they unwittingly are made to contribute to a project of which they disapprove.

Another way in which some subjects may be offended—and have their autonomy violated—if they are used in research without their knowledge or consent is if the study reveals confidential information about them to people they do not want to have it.

This problem can arise even if the patients in the study have data about them collected without any identifiers. One problem arises when the publication of the results reveals that all or virtually all of the subjects had certain characteristics that may be stigmatizing. For example, if the study found that 100% of the users of the clinic where Ms. Arnold's son's teacher was under care had HIV seropositivity, anyone reading that study would know confidential information about him even though he was not named.

The second way that confidence can be broken even though identifiers are not collected is that at the least the one collecting the data sees that patient's chart. Sometimes, as in this case, the data collector may know the patient personally and learn confidential information. In other cases patients may not even want strangers to see their records for some reason. A record search of psychiatric records in a sexual deviancy clinic would raise that possibility. What should be done to protect these patients' right to confidentiality?

In Chapter 7 we saw that the right to confidentiality is sometimes grounded in the principle of fidelity and the duty to keep promises—implied or explicit. Is such a promise made with regard to medical records? Does it apply to examination of the records by a researcher for legitimate scientific purposes?

The *Code of Ethics* of the American Health Information Management Association addresses what it takes to be Ms. Arnold's obligations of confidentiality. It begins by committing the health information professional to confidentiality, but then, in providing detail in its official interpretation, says that the health information management professional should "ensure within his/her scope of responsibility that *all patient identifiable* information will be kept confidential.[20] It also specifies that release of information should be in accordance with current laws and regulations and institutional practices.[21] This raises a potential problem. It is possible that record searches such as the one contemplated by Ms. Arnold are within the letter of the law and conform to institutional policy. If so, is that sufficient for the search to be ethically justified as long as the information is collected without identifying information? Could Ms. Arnold conclude, in effect, that no statement she or her professional group have made conveys or implies that records will not be used in this manner?

Even if health information management professionals can be said not to have promised confidentiality, the problem still exists for other allied health professionals. The American Speech-Language-Hearing Association, for example, explicitly states in its statement on "Ethics in Research and Professional Practice" that "individuals shall use persons in research or as subjects of teaching demonstrations only with their informed consent."[22] No exception is made to permit their members to search records for research purposes when subjects cannot be identified or when the law permits. Can it be that whether it is ethical for an allied health professional to search records without consent depends on which professional group one belongs to?

Perhaps the problem raised by this case can be overcome by an explicit statement given to the patient at the time of admission stating that records will be made available to researchers for research purposes. Or is the right of the patient to confidentiality more fundamental—such that an explicit clarification that the hospital is not promising such broad confidentiality would be unethical?

Another way of arguing that the patient has a right to confidentiality in this case is to appeal to the principle of autonomy. Does autonomy give the patient the right to control the use of his medical records and exclude research uses without explicit consent?

One approach to this problem used by some IRBs involves, first, a statement in the admission consent form that specifies that records (as well as body wastes, remaindered blood, and other products without value to the patient) may be used for research without the patient's consent. Signing the admission consent simultaneously grants approval of the research without further consent. It can be called an "uninformed" or "blank-check" consent.

As long as its use is limited to records, wastes, and the like, this might avoid the violation of autonomy. However, there is a problem. Even patients who generally have no objection to their records being searched for research purposes or their body wastes being studied may occasionally find some element of some specific study objectionable. They might object to the purpose or, as in this case, might object to certain sensitive records being searched. To overcome this problem some IRBs have adopted the policy of treating all research of this sort, which is legally exempt from IRB review, as what is called "expedited" review research. Expedited review is a device by which certain protocol reviews, such as minor changes in the methods, can be reviewed by a single committee member or subcommittee. Only if the reviewer sees a significant problem will the protocol be taken to the entire committee. Would that approach be sufficient to protect patients in cases such as Ms. Arnold's?

In opposition to the concerns about protecting the patient's right of confidentiality is the concern for the good of the society, a good that presumably will be served if research is conducted in an efficient manner. The ethical principle that would support such efforts is normally beneficence, the principle we examined in the cases of Chapter 3. Utilitarians would argue that, in principle, if significant good can be done by the research, then the rights of subjects can be overridden. Is the subject's right to confidentiality such a right that if the good were great enough the investigator could have access even if the subject would object?

EQUITY IN RESEARCH

In the previous case we saw that the ethical principles of fidelity and autonomy might be relevant in assessing research protocols. Even if there is no risk of physical harm to the subject, he could still have his right to confidentiality threatened in ways that could plausibly cause concern. He could also have his right-to-consent to the purpose of the research threatened. Another ethical principle that can sometimes place limits on pursuit of social benefits of research is the principle of justice.

The importance of the principle of justice in assessing medical research involving human subjects has been discovered quite recently. A report of a federal government commission called the *Belmont Report* was the first to mention justice with regard to research.[23]

There are two areas in which questions of justice can arise in research involving human subjects. The one that has received the most attention is subject selection. We have begun to realize that certain groups of people have tended to be particularly vulnerable to being asked to be research subjects. These are often persons who themselves are generally oppressed: the lower-income, ward patients who have very limited options in getting care or prisoners who have even fewer options.

More recently, questions of justice or equity have been raised in the design and conduct of the research. If poorly off people are recruited as subjects—perhaps because they are the only ones who have the condition being studied—some people are claiming that they also have claims of justice to make sure that the research is designed in ways that are as a beneficial as possible to them. For example, instead of making seriously ill patients come to the hospital for tests needed in a protocol, justice may require sending a nurse to their home, making it as easy as possible on them to participate. Some studies have even had their designs modified—reducing the number of tests or the length of the study—to help protect particularly ill research subjects. The case in this section poses the question of the ethics of equity in subject selection.

CASE 70: Equity in Subject Selection

Eastern Hospital is located in a large urban area. Eastern also is a clinical affiliate of a somewhat prestigious medical school. The medical school maintains the clinical affiliation with Eastern so that medical students can obtain an orientation to the patients and problems of a large urban area.

Dr. Dempsey Strong, a young physician who has a specialty in radiotherapy, is an assistant professor with the medical school. He is very dedicated to his work with the college and wants very much to be tenured. He has devised a research project that is administered intraoperatively, that is, during an operation. In this process, radiotherapy can be administered directly to the site that is malignant.

Marceline Train is a young radiotherapist who is working in Eastern Hospital. In just a few years she has risen to become the chief technologist. Dr. Strong has requested that Ms. Train assist him in the research. The protocol that Dr. Strong is employing calls for random participation of consenting patients. One of the variables that is to be studied is the impact of the intraoperative radiotherapy regime on African-American patients. Eastern's patient population is 95% African-American, so it is an ideal site to recruit subjects.

In discussing his protocol with Ms. Train, Dr. Strong indicates that all the African-American patients to be included in the study are to come from Eastern Hospital. Ms. Train, having some knowledge of research protocols (she is a doctoral student in a local university), asks Dr. Strong if his procedure for selection of subjects does not violate the random selection process that is supposed to be employed. She also wonders to herself whether conducting the study is unfair. She sees no reason, in principle, why the study needs to be done on African-American patients (other than that patients at this hospital, which serves largely low-income patients with relatively few options, might make it easier for Dr. Strong to get subjects). Does the study violate the requirement of equity in subject selection, and should Ms. Train object on these grounds?

The regulatory requirement that subjects must be selected equitably is rather new. It poses what may often be a direct conflict between the principle of justice, which requires distributing the benefits and burdens of the research enterprise fairly, and the principle of beneficence, which requires that the investigator maximize the benefit he can be expected to produce.

Researchers have long gravitated to vulnerable, low-income populations for their research subjects. They have been easier to recruit, perhaps believing that if they do not cooperate, they will not get needed medical care. They are believed to ask fewer questions and comply more readily with the investigator's requests.

If this is true, then recruiting such subjects is an efficient way in which to conduct research. It is not only permitted, but mandated by the principle of beneficence (unless, of course, such a policy would produce a backlash jeopardizing the research enterprise). Thus, Ms. Train has encountered what may well be a direct conflict between the principles of justice and beneficence. The issue here is how the two competing claims can be reconciled.

The federal regulations require that a series of criteria be satisfied for a study to be approved by the IRB. These include the requirement that the study produce benefits to society that justify the risks as well as those that confidentiality be protected, consent be obtained, and equity in subject selection be satisfied.

The ethical question is whether each of these must be satisfied before a research project is considered ethically acceptable. Must consent, confidentiality, and selection equity all be fully assured before Dr. Strong can turn to his claim that significant benefits can be expected from completing his study? Or do these earlier requirements (grounded in autonomy, fidelity, and justice) enter into a compromise with beneficence so that if the expected results are believed to be quite valuable, certain liberties can be taken with consent, confidentiality, or equity? Should Ms. Train insist that subjects be recruited equitably from other more affluent hospitals as well as Eastern? Should she ask the IRB to reassess its approval on the grounds that equity in subject selection is not assured?

INFORMED CONSENT IN RESEARCH

In the two previous cases, the requirements of confidentiality and equity in subject selection—grounded in the principles of fidelity to promises and justice—provided reasons why some would place limits on research even if it is believed to be well designed and is likely to produce significant benefits for the society. These two ethical principles not focusing on maximizing good consequences potentially could hold social beneficence in check, protecting the rights of patients even though societal benefits might be lost in the process.

Another way in which societal interests come into conflict with the moral requirements of other principles of ethics is in the area of informed consent. As we saw in Chapter 5, the consent requirement is often grounded in autonomy rather than utility. Consent is required according to the principle of autonomy, even if the health professional believes that more benefit to the patient or society might result if the consent requirements were ignored.

This conflict between autonomy and social benefit arises frequently in cases in which investigators believe that the consent should be waived or modified to assure greater benefit for the society from the research. The next case illustrates the problem.

CASE 71: Informed Consent in Research

Nancy Lowe is a physical therapist who works in a pain management clinic. The clinic has received a federal grant to explore the effectiveness of transcutaneous electrical stimulation (TENS) for treatment of low-back pain. The research protocol calls for four options to be explored, including TENS with hotpacks, TENS with ice, ice alone, and hotpacks alone. Her protocol calls for randomizing her patients to one of these four treatments.

Since hotpacks, ice, and transcutaneous electrical stimulation are normally employed in the treatment of persons with low-back pain, the investigators believe that the research protocol does not need to include informed consent, but does require approximately an equal number of patients to be assigned to each of the four treatment options just noted.

Nancy Lowe also decides to forgo the informed consent with the research project because patients when given a choice will always elect to avoid ice treatment. Most people feel that ice is too uncomfortable.

Donald Taylor, a construction worker, has injured his back on the job. When he comes in for treatment at the pain management clinic, Mr. Taylor is assigned to have ice and TENS. He inquires of Nancy Lowe if he has a choice. How should she respond?

Ms. Lowe seems to assume that as long as she is conducting a randomized trial of four treatments, all of which are standard treatments in clinical use, she is under no obligation to obtain Mr. Taylor's informed consent. That assumption is not warranted. Assuming that Ms. Lowe is conducting a piece of research designed to produce generalizable knowledge, she is involved in some interventions that have purposes unrelated the normal therapy. For example, the randomization itself is not part of her standard treatment; it is a research intervention. Moreover, she will record data, perhaps asking her patients questions about how well the treatment is doing, maybe using a standardized questionnaire. None of these are part of standard therapy. As long as there are research interventions designed to produce generalizable knowledge (whether it will be published or not), most commentators would hold that a research consent is required.

Getting that consent may be inconvenient for Ms. Lowe. Sometimes investigators defend ignoring the consent on the grounds that patients would not object as long as all the treatments are standard. Does such an argument or the worry about the inconvenience of having to get consent justify waiving the consent in this case? The current federal government guidelines specify that under special circumstances, the consent can be waived, provided the risks are minimal (presumably they are here). But three other conditions must also be met. First, there must be no other way that the study could be conducted. Second, the subjects must be debriefed afterward (telling them the nature of the research and why they were not asked to consent in the first place). Can Ms. Lowe meet either of these conditions? Finally, the regulations say that if consent is to be omitted, the rights of the subject must not be adversely affected."[24]

This poses a paradox. It is often held that one of the rights of the subject is to consent to participate in research. If that is one of the rights of subjects, the only cases in which consent could be waived are those in which the right-to-consent has been respected.

There is a further problem facing Ms. Lowe. One of the core ethical premises of randomized clinical trials is that the null hypothesis must be plausible; that is, the hypothesis that there is no difference among the treatments must be sincerely believable. (Otherwise, the treatment that cannot be believed to be comparable must be excluded from the trial.) The investigator must be at what can be called the "indifference point," that is, the point at which one is more or less indifferent among the treatment options. It is only ethical to conduct a trial if there is legitimate doubt as to which treatment is better.

That poses a problem for Ms. Lowe. She, herself, claims that if she gave people a choice, they would refuse the ice because it is "too uncomfortable." If she acknowledges that one of her treatments would be rejected by a significant number of patients, she will have a hard time honestly maintaining that one should be indifferent among the options. Of course, she might believe that there are possible advantages to the use of the ice that would just offset the discomfort. In that case the net potential benefits might be comparable to the other treatment options, and she could legitimately be indifferent. If that were the case, however, she would have to be able to explain this indifference to patients. Moreover, just because she and other competent physical therapists believe that the potential benefits balance the discomfort, that does not mean all her patients will balance the two in the same way. We have seen in earlier chapters that assessing benefits and risks is inherently a subjective process. Different people will make the assessments differently. Mr. Taylor may not quantify the potential benefits or the discomfort of the ice the same way Ms. Lowe does. He may rationally believe that the other options are better even if Ms. Lowe really is indifferent.

This poses an even more serious problem for Ms. Lowe. She seems to believe that if this were not part of a research project, there would be no question of her getting consent from her patients for the treatment. That raises the question of informed consent for therapeutic medicine, the topic of the cases in the next chapter.

Before turning to that chapter, consider Ms. Lowe's situation. She apparently has four treatments to choose from and is legitimately perplexed about which is better. Presumably any one of them would be an accepted treatment. Yet it is precisely in such situations that, under the principle of autonomy, patients should be informed of their options and permitted to choose among the plausible options. It may be that whether Ms. Lowe considers her intervention research or therapy, she has a consent problem. It is to the role of consent in therapy that we now turn.

ENDNOTES

1. "Nuremberg Code, 1946," in *Encyclopedia of Bioethics*, Vol. 4, ed. Warren T. Reich (New York: The Free Press, 1978), pp. 1764-1765.
2. American Physical Therapy Association, *Guide for Professional Conduct* Alexandria, VA: APTA, July 1994).
3. The American Dietetic Association, *Code of Ethics for the Profession of Dietetics and Review Process for Alleged Violations* (Chicago: ADA, 1988).
4. American Academy of Physician Assistants, *Code of Ethics of the Physician Assistant Profession* (Alexandria, VA: AAPA, adopted 1983, amended 1985 House of Delegates).
5. American Speech-Language-Hearing Association, *Code of Ethics*, published in *Asha*, Vol. 34 (March 1992), Suppl. 9, pp. 1-2.
6. "Nuremberg Code, 1946," in *Encyclopedia of Bioethics*, Vol. 4, pp. 1764-1765, point 2 of the code, ed. Warren T. Reich (New York: The Free Press, 1978).
7. Ibid., point 1 of code.
8. World Medical Association, "Declaration of Helsinki—1964," in *Encyclopedia of Bioethics*, Vol. 4, ed. by Warren T. Reich (New York: The Free Press, 1978), pp. 1769-1771.
9. Ibid., Part III, point 3a.
10. American Medical Association, *Ethical Guidelines for Clinical Investigation*, in *Encyclopedia of Bioethics*, Vol. 4, pp. 1773-1774.
11. American Occupational Therapy Association, *Occupational Therapy Code of Ethics*, published in *American Journal of Occupational Therapy*, Vol. 42 (December 1988), pp. 795-796.
12. American Speech-Language-Hearing Association (ASLHA), *Ethics in Research and Professional Practice*, published in *Asha*, Vol. 34 (March 1992), Suppl. 9, pp. 11-12; American Physical Therapy Association, *Guide for Professional Conduct* (Alexandria, VA: APTA, July 1991).
13. U.S. Department of Health, Education, and Welfare, *The Institutional Guide to DHEW Policy on Protection of Human Subjects* (Washington, DC: U.S. Government Printing Office, 1971).
14. U.S. Department of Health and Human Services, "Final Regulations Amending Basic HHS Policy for the Protection of Human Research Subjects: Final Rule: 45 CFR 46," *Federal Register: Rules and Regulations*, Vol. 46, no. 16 (January 26, 1981), pp. 8366-8392.

15. U.S. Department of Health and Human Services (USDHHS), "Federal Policy for the Protection of Human Subjects: Notices and Rules," *Federal Register*, Vol. 46, no. 117 (June 18, 1991), pp. 28001-28032.
16. American Speech-Language-Hearing Association, *Code of Ethics of the American Speech-Language-Hearing Association* (Rockville, MD: ASLHA, January 1, 1990), p. 1.
17. ASLHA, *Ethics in Research and Professional Practice*.
18. U.S. Department of Health and Human Services, "Federal Policy for the Protection of Human Subjects: Notices and Rules," *Federal Register*, Vol. 46, no. 117 (June 18, 1991), pp. 28015-28016.
19. U.S. Department of Health and Human Services, "Federal Policy for the Protection of Human Subjects; Notices and Rules," *Federal Register*, Vol. 46, no. 117 (June 18, 1991), p. 28012.
20. American Medical Records Association, *AMRA Code of Ethics: Guide to the Interpretation of the Code of Ethics*—1985 Revision, published in *Journal of AMRA* (October 1987), p. 57.
21. Ibid.
22. ASLHA, *Ethics in Research and Professional Practice*, p. 12.
23. National Commission for the Protection of Human Subjects of Biomedical and Behavioral Research, *The Belmont Report: Ethical Principles and Guidelines for the Protection of Human Subjects of Research* (Washington, DC: U.S. Government Printing Office, 1978).
24. USDHHS, "Federal Policy for the Protection of Human Subjects," p. 28017.

CHAPTER 13

Consent and the Right to Refuse Treatment

Issues of informed consent that arise in medical research were discussed in the final case of the previous chapter. Informed consent has also emerged as a central issue in therapeutic medicine, at least in the last half of the twentieth century.[1]

It is striking that the Hippocratic ethical tradition has no provision for consent of the patient for any treatment. Its central ethical approach was to assume that the physician could figure out what was in the interest of the patient and act accordingly. The Hippocratic Oath actually prohibits the health care professional from sharing any medical knowledge with patients.[2]

It was not until the twentieth century that consent of the patient became morally important. Its moral foundation is generally not in the moral principles of doing good and protecting from harm, but in the key principle of Western political philosophy: self-determination or autonomy. As we saw in Chapter 5, autonomy as a moral principle requires that people be allowed to make life choices according to self-generated life plans. In medicine this means consenting to health care choices that fit with one's own goals and purposes.

The realization that different health care choices will be appropriate for different life plans is one of the most revolutionary in the health care ethics of the twentieth century. At first, the only requirement was that the patient actually agree to the treatment. A key legal case in 1914 summarized the emerging notion saying, "Every human being of adult years and sound mind has a right to determine what shall be done with his own body; and a surgeon who performs an operation without his patient's consent commits an assault, for which he is liable in damages."[3]

We gradually began to realize that it was possible for a patient to consent to treatment and still not be informed about the choices being made. It was not until the 1950s that concern began to emerge that consent be informed and voluntary.[4] That introduced several important questions in the discussion of consent. In the first section of this chapter, we shall look at what can be called the *elements of consent*, that is, the types of information that need to be transmitted for a consent to be adequately informed. In the second section, we shall look at cases involving questions of the *standards of consent*. This refers to the question of what standard of reference should be used in determining whether a sufficient amount of a particular type of information has been transmitted. In the third section we shall examine the questions of whether the information transmitted is comprehended and whether the consent is adequately voluntary. Here is the place where we shall address whether incompetent patients can be expected to consent and what role parents, guardians, and other surrogates can play in giving approval of medical treatments for those who are legally incompetent to do so themselves.

THE ELEMENTS OF A CONSENT

An adequate consent to treatment must be informed. For it to be informed it must contain several types of information, not only information about the benefits and harms, but also their probabilities of occurring as well as information about treatment alternatives. There may be other kinds of information that patients would desire as well, including information about the costs of the treatment, inconvenience, the time consumed, risks relating to confidentiality breaches, and the competence of the provider. The following cases show how allied health professionals may face problems in deciding whether patients have been given enough information for their consent to be adequately informed.

CASE 72: Is Death a Risk Worth Discussing or Is It a Benefit?

William Tendler is a respiratory care practitioner who has worked the medical intensive care unit for the past three years. He has seen many patients whose lives were saved by his aggressive care, but he has also seen patients who run a great risk of becoming respirator-dependent, stranded on ventilators.

Eighty-six-year-old Gertrude Stewart has been hospitalized in the ICU for the past 12 days following a stroke. She is now conscious and somewhat alert, but unable to walk, talk, or breathe on her own. She is maintained on a ventilator, which Mr. Tendler supervises. She is able to communicate with motion of her head. She seems to understand simple questions and answers coherently.

When Mrs. Stewart arrived at the hospital, she was unable to communicate at all. Support, including the ventilator, was started on an emergency basis. Later, her daughter, Mary Kline, who is age 57, was informed of the steps being taken.

Mr. Tendler was present during that conversation. It was clear that Dr. Benson, the attending physician, had not discussed the chances of successful recovery with Mrs. Kline nor with the patient. Mr. Tendler confirmed this from the medical record and from conversations with the head nurse. While reviewing the record Mr. Tendler discovered that Mrs. Stewart had been coded DNR, or "do not resuscitate," in the event of a cardiac or respiratory arrest.

When Mr. Tendler asked Dr. Benson about how much Mrs. Stewart and her daughter knew about the situation, Dr. Benson indicated that he had assessed Mrs. Stewart's condition and had made the choices that he thought were in her interest. He wanted to continue her on the ventilator because he thought there was some chance she could be weaned and returned to an active life. On the other hand, he believed that, should she suffer a cardiac arrest, the compounding of the present damage with the new assault would make matters hopeless for her.

Mr. Tendler pressed him about whether Mrs. Stewart or her daughter should be consulted about these choices. Dr. Benson took offense, saying, "The single most important thing a physician can do for a patient is protect her from harm. She has to be spared the agony of a bleak prognosis. Moreover, if she were told about the low possibility of being weaned from the ventilator, she would surely become discouraged and might even irrationally try to get the ventilator disconnected."

Mr. Tendler is not convinced with Dr. Benson's reasoning. He realizes that at some point in the near future, he will be providing maintenance for the ventilator. It seems to him that the present support constitutes treatment without informed consent. He is likely to be the one Mrs. Stewart or her daughter asks to stop the treatment. Also, if she arrests, he would be directly involved in resuscitating or standing by withholding the CPR. He also realizes that were he to resuscitate her, he would be treating not only against the physician's order, but possibly against the patient's will. On the other hand, if he follows the DNR order, he will be directly contributing to her death in a manner that she might not want.

Mr. Tendler realizes that there are good reasons why reasonable people would disagree over exactly where to draw the line. The doctrine of informed consent requires that information must be disclosed to the patient (or her surrogate) that she reasonably would need to know to choose whether to authorize treatment. (We will discuss, in the next section of this chapter, what standards should be used in deciding exactly how much information needs to be transmitted. For now, the critical issues are what are the elements of a consent and what kinds of information must be transmitted.)

The benefits of the ventilator and the anticipated CPR are perhaps obvious. But there is every reason to believe that neither Mrs. Stewart nor her daughter really knows what the possible outcomes are or the chances of those outcomes occurring. The concept of ventilator dependency is one not ordinarily in the working vocabulary of most patients. If Mrs. Stewart is to be adequately informed, certainly she should know the likely outcomes and their probability, expressed in at least general terms. She also needs to know what would usually be called the side effects: the respirator dependency, the likelihood of partial recovery of function, the frustrations of a clouded mental function, and the like. With regard to the anticipated CPR, she should know something about the likelihood of success and what the clinician considers a success. None of these seems to have been made available to her.

There are other pieces of information that she might have use for: the costs of the treatment, how much insurance is covering, and whether there are treatment alternatives available (nursing homes, home care programs, physical therapy, and more aggressive treatment options). The fact that there are others, both within the health care team and outside of it, who might have different views about what the best course is, might also be an element of a consent process that should be conveyed to the patient. Are there other kinds of information that could be conveyed to this patient or her daughter?

Many controversies over what information to transmit to a patient focus on benefits and harms of the proposed treatment or alternatives. Sometimes, however, for a consent to be adequately informed, the patient may have to be given others kinds of information. The patient may need to know about the cost of the treatment or inconvenience related to administration. In other cases the risk that might be disclosed pertains to the competence of the provider or the institution. Even if the treatment in competent hands might be perfectly acceptable to the patient, the same treatment might give the patient pause in the hands of certain providers. The following case illustrates the problem.

CASE 73: Conflict Within the Team

Shirley Monson, an occupational therapist who is employed by the Carter Rehabilitation Center, is working with David Dillard, a patient who has quadriplegia due to what was diagnosed as a C5-6 spinal cord lesion. During the course of therapy, Ms. Monson notices that his function is improving and that he is gaining some skills expected only with a lower-level lesion (C7-8). This particular patient's physician is paternalistic and authoritarian in his interactions with patients and staff. The physician has stated that this patient will achieve function expected with a C5-6 lesion and has set the goals for therapy accordingly.

The physician is preparing to discharge the patient from the center since all goals have been met. The physical therapist and the nurse are in agreement. The occupational therapist wants to extend the patient's stay to allow him to achieve maximum independence in dressing. She believes he can move from his present status of needing moderate physical assistance to dress in bed to the point where he will need minimal or standby assistance.

Ms. Monson realizes that part of an informed consent is an explanation of the alternatives to the therapy proposed. Ms. Monson believes that Mr. Dillard should be told that an alternative to the therapy based on the assumption of a C5-6 lesion would be to treat this as a C7-8 lesion. She wonders whether she should do something about what Mr. Dillard has been told, which she believes is inadequate. She also wonders whether part of the consent process in this case should include informing the patient that part of the health care team believes there may have been an error in the diagnosis.

Ms. Monson probably realizes that doubts about the adequacy of the diagnosis and disagreements among members of the health care team about the therapeutic plan are not normally part of the consent process. Still, she faces a choice about the consent. If the purpose of the consent process is to facilitate patient autonomy, as was suggested in Chapter 5, then in cases like this one perhaps the most important information the patient could have in making autonomous choices is information about the occupational therapist's doubts about the diagnosis and limits on the therapy.

The other members of the health care team seem to agree with the physician's view. Under these circumstances, what should the occupational therapist do? One approach would be to talk with her colleagues. Assuming they continue to believe that the physician's judgment is correct and are unwilling to challenge this authoritarian practitioner, what other options are available to Ms. Monson? Should she speak to her supervisor who, in turn, could talk with the physician or the director of the rehabilitation service? to the patient himself? Is Mr. Dillard's consent adequately informed without this information? A similar problem arises in the next case.

CASE 74: Informed Consent and an Incompetent Physician

Anne Burgess has had 10 years of experience as a hand therapist. A patient, Luther Siemer, is referred by John Lanham, a surgeon who has never referred his patients before. This patient was involved in a car accident in which his hand was pinned under a car, causing multiple fractures. Dr. Lanham has given orders that therapy be initiated to increase active range of motion and strength.

Ms. Burgess evaluates the patient during the first therapy session and looks at the x-rays, which were taken after surgery. She realizes that the surgery was done incorrectly. The pins do not hit the fracture sites, the fractured bones are not properly aligned, the hand is out of alignment in general, and the splint that was made by the surgeon is not providing proper support. Nonetheless, the patient states that he is pleased with the results. She knows that with his hand in this condition, the therapy to increase the active range of motion and strengthening is contraindicated.

Ms. Burgess normally assumes that consent for physical therapy is implied by the fact that the patient shows up and begins the therapy. Any questions, she presumes, are answered by the referring physician, but now she realizes that this patient lacks some important information: that a member of the health care team believes the surgeon has not provided an adequate procedure. She also realizes that she may be the only one who could inform the patient of the dangers of providing the prescribed therapy. What does she do about the inadequate consent?

As with the previous case, the therapist realizes that the consent may be inadequate. For one thing, she realizes that there is a significant risk of harm if the therapy is provided as prescribed.

Some health care providers might ask whether physical therapy is a treatment that needs consent. That way of putting the question assumes that there are some procedures that need consent and others that do not. In fact, that is not correct. All procedures need consent in some form. Some of them may involve procedures so well understood by the patient that the consent can be said to be presumed or implied. In effect, we can say in such cases that the patient is adequately informed just based on general knowledge and common sense. Nothing explicit needs to be said for the patient to give an adequate consent. However, there may be special circumstances involving even the most routine procedures in which the patient may need some information. In this case, there is a serious risk that the patient cannot suspect. The risk appears to be of such importance that the patient cannot possibly be said to have consented to the treatment unless he is told.

Had Ms. Burgess consulted the code of ethics of the American Physical Therapy Association, she might have been surprised and somewhat confused with what she found. First, the code nowhere commits the physical therapist to getting informed consent from patients, either implicitly or explicitly. In the "Guide for Professional Conduct," which expands on the code, there are two references to consent, but neither has anything directly to do with consenting to treatment. The first (Principle 1.2.A) commits the therapist who is a member of the association to getting consent before releasing confidential information. The second (Principle 4.3.B) requires consent for research on human subjects. Neither deals with consent to nonexperimental therapy. That having been said, there are hints in the code that Ms. Burgess may be expected by her professional association to disclose the situation she faces. Principle 3.1.B seems relevant. It requires that "When the individual's needs are beyond the scope of the physical therapist's expertise, or when additional services are indicated, the individual shall be so informed and assisted in identifying a qualified provider."[5] That mandate applied to Ms. Burgess' case would leave her in an awkward spot, presumably informing her patient that what he needs is "beyond the scope of her expertise." Moreover, in the next paragraph, the physical therapist is told that "When physical therapists judge that benefit can no longer be obtained from their services, they shall so inform the individual receiving the services. It is unethical to continue or initiate services that, in the therapist's judgement, either cannot result in beneficial outcome or are contraindicated." Following these provisions may, in effect, have the same implications as requiring that consent be obtained for the prescribed services. Either way, presumably, the patient is informed of the inappropriate treatment and declines to proceed. The code may actually go further in requiring that the therapist not proceed.

What options are open to Ms. Burgess assuming she is convinced that she cannot treat this patient without an explicit consent and that Mr. Siemer has to be told about her belief that the treatment was wrong?

From the three cases presented in this section, it would appear that among the elements of consent that must be conveyed for a consent to be informed are the anticipated benefits and risks of the procedure and their probabilities, alternative treatments available, costs of treatment and the alternatives, and the clinician's concern about the competence and ability of other members of the health care team. In some cases, there may be other elements such as research or financial interests that might influence the provider, the nature of disagreements among the health care team, and other information that could be useful to the patient in deciding for or against treatment.

Once the categories or elements of information are understood, there still remains the question of just how much information must be provided. This requires assessment of the alternative standards for consent.

THE STANDARDS FOR CONSENT

In the previous section we saw that there were elements of information that could be part of a consent—such as the competence of the provider—that are normally not told to patients that nevertheless are potentially very important in some cases. Probably if allied health professionals asked their colleagues—fellow professionals and members of the other professions—they would find that their colleagues in similar situations often would not disclose this potentially important information. This practice of nondisclosure raises an important question: Should the consensus of one's colleagues be the standard for deciding what must be disclosed?

Deciding what to disclose based on what one's colleagues would disclose is what is called the *professional standard*. Traditional legal and moral practice relied on the professional standard for determining what must be disclosed.

Beginning about 1970 our standard began to change. There emerged what is now called the *reasonable person standard*.[6] It replaces the idea that one is required to disclose what one's colleagues similarly situated would have disclosed with the idea that one is required to disclose what the reasonable person would want or need to know to make an informed choice for or against the proposed treatment.

The argument is that if the goal is to give information needed in order to make autonomous choices, then it really is not decisive what professional colleagues similarly situated would disclose. They may also have developed a practice that does not provide the patient with everything he or she wants or needs to know. Only telling what one needs to know will do the job.

The reasonable person standard makes a controversial presumption: that what the "reasonable person" would need is what a particular patient would need. But what about the patient who is unique, who would like some information that the typical reasonable person would not want? Or what about the patient who is unique in not wanting some information that the typical reasonable person would need? Some are now proposing a *subjective standard*.[7] It would require disclosing what the actual patient would want or need to know rather than either what colleagues would disclose or what the reasonable person would need to know. The following case requires the allied health professional to choose which of these three standards is appropriate.

CASE 75: But My Colleagues Wouldn't Tell Either

John Wills is a radiation therapist in a large city hospital. He recently reported a situation he felt was very disturbing. Dr. Cindy Adams, the specialist in radiation therapy, had referred Mr. James Cell to the clinic for therapy. Mr. Cell reports that he was very apprehensive about going to the clinic for the radiation; however, Dr. Adams told him it would only take about five minutes.

When Mr. Wills received the orders, he noted that Mr. Cell was to have the radiation therapy applied to several sites. By the time the therapy was completed, Mr. Cell was in the clinic for 90 minutes—a far cry from the 5 minutes that had been promised by Dr. Adams.

In talking with his supervisor, John Wills indicated that he was quite upset with Dr. Adams. He was not upset with the patient in this instance. "She should have known that a five minute treatment was out of the question."

When queried by her supervisor, Dr. Adams indicated that she was aware of Mr. Cell's apprehension. She insisted that she told Mr. Cell only what her other physician colleagues would tell an apprehensive patient. She had intentionally misled him because she thought it would increase the chance he would get the treatment he needed.

Mr. Wills was also concerned about the fact that Dr. Adams only indicated to Mr. Cell that there would be one treatment site when in fact there were three. Mr. Wills wondered if Mr. Cell would have given his consent to the treatment if he had known that there were three treatment sites. Again, Dr. Adams responded that she handles the multiple sites issue in the same way that her physician colleagues do. According to her, it was "just standard practice."

The issues raised in this case can be analyzed as an informed consent problem. Normally, informing a patient in the process of getting consent for treatment includes telling the patient the risks as well as the benefits. It also includes telling the patient the alternatives. While the risks might be thought of as the possible undesired physical consequences of the treatment, such as radiation burns, mutations of cells, or other undesired effects, they might also include such things as a true account of the time that will be involved, the number of sites to be radiated, and the like. Sometimes the psychological stress of the treatment or the inconvenience might also be part of what reasonable people would want to know. Is it reasonable to expect that Mr. Cell would want to know about the time involved and the number of sites?

This case can also be analyzed under the rubric of the principle of veracity or truth-telling. In Chapter 6 the cases introduced the problem of whether there is a moral duty to be honest with the patient in cases in which the physician believes it is contrary to the patient's interest. Here Dr. Adams seemed to believe that Mr. Cell would be hurt in some way if he were told the truth. What evidence is there that he would be hurt? Is there reason to believe he would have refused the radiation had he known of the length of time and the number of sites?

Assuming that he would have refused the radiation, Dr. Adams probably believed this would be bad for him. The moral principles of autonomy and veracity require that the patient be permitted to accept or refuse an offered treatment after having been informed truthfully about the relevant information. On the other hand, holders of the primacy of the principle of beneficence sometimes claim that the physician has a duty to benefit the patient even if it means violating autonomy or veracity. Which principle should win out here?

Assuming that there is a duty to get an informed consent in such cases, Dr. Adams must realize that she cannot tell Mr. Cell literally everything about the radiation treatment. There are virtually infinite effects that could occur, many of which he clearly would not be interested in learning about. There is no way she can tell him *everything*. Knowing what to disclose depends on which standard is appropriate. According to the traditional professional standard, Dr. Adams need tell only what her colleagues similarly situated would have claimed. She claims, probably correctly, that other physicians would not have disclosed all the details about the time involved. If she can show that her colleagues would not have said any more, is that a sufficient defense of her actions?

The reasonable person standard holds that she must tell what the reasonable person would want to know before consenting. Would the reasonable person want to know that the time involved was 90 minutes rather than 5 minutes? Would he or she want to know there were three sites rather than one? If so, then by the reasonable person standard, Dr. Adams would have to disclose. The moral principle behind this reasonable person standard is autonomy: the patient must be told what he or she needs to know to make an informed choice even if the information will be upsetting.

Of course, Mr. Cell was not a typical patient. He was unusually apprehensive about the radiation. Dr. Adams seemed to know that; that is the justification she used for not disclosing the true nature of the procedure. In such cases, to promote autonomy, the physician might have to meet the subjective standard, by which the physician must disclose what the particular patient would want to know, even if that differs from what the typical reasonable person would want. Would Mr. Cell want more or less information than the reasonable person?

Applying the subjective standard poses serious problems. It is clear that the clinician cannot be held responsible for knowing all the ways in which the patient has unique desires about information. The subjective standard does require, however, that the clinician inform the patient based on the patient's own desires and values when the clinician knows them or should be expected to know them. This might, for instance, be based on the clinician's general knowledge of the interests and personality of the patient. It might also be furthered by asking the patient, in an open and encouraging way, whether he has any special concerns or questions. Otherwise, the clinician can revert to the more objective reasonable person standard. It is the obligation of the patient to let the clinician know unique concerns, as Mr. Cell apparently did in this case.

COMPREHENSION AND VOLUNTARINESS

It is not enough that the patient be adequately informed if the consent is to satisfy the requirements of the principle of autonomy. The information must also be understood, and the consent must be voluntary. Consent may be constrained either because the information, though communicated, was not understood or because the individual's choice was somehow not voluntary.

Understanding is jeopardized when the words cannot be comprehended because they are unfamiliar—either because the patient is not a native speaker or, even if he or she is a native speaker, the terms are simply too complex. Psychological factors, such as stress from an illness, may also make the information incomprehensible.

Even if the patient understands, the consent may not be voluntary. The patient can be constrained externally by undue physical or psychological pressures or internally by mental illness or compulsion. The following case raises the problem of whether a consent is based on adequate comprehension and voluntariness.

CASE 76: Too Confused to Be Informed?

Olivia Morgan, a 65-year-old, moderately retarded, widowed woman who recently underwent a mastectomy, has reported to the physical therapy clinic for treatment. The area where the surgery occurred has been desensitized. She had been quite disturbed by the diagnosis of breast cancer and the surgery she had undergone. It left her even more confused. Mrs. Morgan has not been totally informed about the heat treatment that she is to receive from Julie Westermann, the clinic physical therapist.

The normal amount of time for which hot packs are to be applied is 20-25 minutes. Patients are supposed to be told that they should report any discomfort to the physical therapist. When Mrs. Morgan reported for therapy, she was not informed about this risk. After approximately 20 minutes of treatment, the pack was removed, but it was discovered that Mrs. Morgan suffered a burn.

Mrs. Morgan was not informed by Ms. Westermann because she believed Mrs. Morgan to be too confused to comprehend the instructions and precautions. When queried about the situation, Mrs. Morgan stated that she felt some pain, but thought that unless there was some pain, the treatment was not doing any good.

Some physical therapy treatments are such routine, low-risk procedures that some physicians and allied health professionals may believe that informed consent is not required. They may believe that consent is only necessary for complex and dangerous procedures such as surgery or experimental therapies. That is a mistake. In fact, if consent has its foundations in autonomy and the goal is to assure that the patient's medical treatment fits within the patient's life plan, then all treatments must require at least some kind of consent. Often consent may be implied (as when a patient extends an arm for drawing blood). It may be presumed as in certain emergencies in which the law authorizes us to presume a patient would want to receive enough treatment to stabilize the patient and permit the patient to make further choices.

If, as was suggested in the previous section, patients cannot be told *everything*, but need to be told only what they want to know in order to offer an adequately informed choice, then some interventions, including some physical therapy, may require only a general explanation in the normal case.

If, however, the patient is at special risk or has particular difficulty understanding, then further steps might have to be taken for the consent to be informed.

Some patients may be believed by the therapist to be so lacking in capacity to comprehend an explanation that they, in fact, are incapable of giving a consent. They are said to lack capacity to consent. A therapist cannot, however, simply conclude unilaterally that this is the case. Doing so would, in effect, be declaring the patient incompetent. That is something that can only be done through the judicial system.

Even if a patient were declared incompetent, as Ms. Westermann may feel is appropriate here, normally a surrogate or guardian must be appointed and that surrogate would have to consent to the treatment.

Ms. Westermann has a problem if she must seek judicial intervention every time she has a patient who she believes cannot comprehend the nature of the procedure and its risks. Fortunately, some patients are presumed legally to be incompetent including children and those who have previously been declared wards of the state. They already have surrogates or guardians capable of speaking for them, and the consent must be obtained from these surrogates.

In other cases, such as Mrs. Morgan's, no formal ruling has declared the patient incompetent. Some people are saying that in such cases, the provider might ask the patient if she is willing to have someone act as a surrogate. If the patient agrees (or if the patient is too disoriented to reply), most clinicians are willing to presume that the patient lacks capacity. If the patient protests, then generally it must be presumed the patient is competent until declared otherwise.

Ms. Westermann still would have a problem. Her patient is an older, unmarried woman who has no readily available surrogate. Moreover, even if she did have a surrogate, it is not clear that the surrogate's consent would solve the problem. In this case it was important for the patient to understand the possibility of the packs being too hot and causing a burn. Merely telling that to a surrogate would not do much good unless the surrogate could communicate this to the patient and urge the patient to report any problem.

Does the lack of capacity on Mrs. Morgan's part justify treating her without consent? Are there steps that Ms. Westermann should have taken to assure that Mrs. Morgan understands the risks of the procedure?

Many of the most controversial informed consent cases involve consent or refusal of consent for treatment for critical or terminal illness. Patients may refuse consent knowing that they may be at risk for dying. In fact, they may actually be wanting to die when they refuse the consent. These issues arise in the cases in Chapter 14.

ENDNOTES

1. President's Commission for the Study of Ethical Problems in Medicine and Biomedical and Behavioral Research, *Making Health Care Decisions: A Report on the Ethical and Legal Implications of Informed Consent in the Patient-Practitioner Relationship*, Vol. 1 (Washington, DC: U.S. Government Printing Office, 1982); Charles W. Lidz, Alan Meisel, Evitar Zerubavel, Mary Carter, Regina M. Sestak, and Loren H. Roth, *Informed Consent: A Study of Decisionmaking in Psychiatry* (New York: The Guilford Press, 1984); Ruth Faden and Tom L. Beauchamp in collaboration with Nancy N. P. King, *A History and Theory of Informed Consent* (New York: Oxford University Press, 1986); Jay Katz, *The Silent World of Doctor and Patient* (New York: The Free Press, 1984).
2. Ludwig Edelstein, "The Hippocratic Oath: Text, Translation and Interpretation," *Ancient Medicine: Selected Papers of Ludwig Edelstein*, eds. Owsei and C. Lilian Temkin (Baltimore, MD: The Johns Hopkins Press, 1967), p. 6 (also see pp. 3-64).
3. *Schloendorff* v. *New York Hospital* (1914), in Jay Katz, *Experimentation with Human Beings: The Authority of the Investigator, Subject, Professions, and State in the Human Experimentation Process* (New York: Russell Sage Foundation, 1972), p. 526.
4. *Salgo* v. *Leland Stanford Jr. University Board of Trustees*, 317 P.2d 170 (1957).
5. American Physical Therapy Association, *Guide for Professional Conduct* (Alexandria, VA: APTA, July 1994).
6. *Berkey* v. *Anderson*, 1 Cal. App. 3d 790. 82 Cal. Rptr. 67 (1969); *Cobbs* v. *Grant*, 502 P.2d 1 (Cal. 1972); *Canterbury* v. *Spence*, U.S. Court of Appeals, District of Columbia, 1972, 464 F.2d 772, 150 U.S. App. D.C. 263.
7. President's Commission for the Study of Ethical Problems in Medicine and Biomedical and Behavioral Research, *Making Health Care Decisions: A Report on the Ethical and Legal Implications of Informed Consent in the Patient-Practitioner Relationship*, Vol. 1 (Washington, DC: U.S. Government Printing Office, 1982), p. 43.

CHAPTER 14

Death and Dying

The informed consent issues raised in the previous chapter often arise in the care of terminally and critically ill patients. In the consent process patients must be told of the treatment alternatives. With terminally ill patients, sometimes doing nothing to attempt a cure is among the plausible alternatives. The terminally ill patient (or his or her surrogate) may decline the treatment offered in favor of letting nature take its course. While this is sometimes referred to as doing nothing at all, in fact it normally involves continuing to care for the patient while forgoing efforts to *cure*. The pioneering medical ethicist Paul Ramsey was one who stressed the distinction between curing and caring and the appropriateness of continuing to care when cure becomes impossible.[1] Others have summarized the moral issues related to terminal care decisions.[2] Often it is the allied health professional staff who have special responsibilities for continuing to care for the dying patient to make him or her comfortable.

In the cases of Chapter 8 the problems surrounding the ethics of killing and letting die were examined. Some traditional medical ethics, such as Orthodox Judaism, include the belief that medical professionals always have a duty to preserve life.[3] We saw in Chapter 8, however, that many medical ethical traditions, including those in the health care professions[4] as well as U.S. law,[5] often distinguish between active killing, which is prohibited, and forgoing treatment, which can legitimately be chosen by the patient or surrogate under certain circumstances. We also saw that deciding what was ethical to forgo is often based on assessment of benefits and harms expected. The doctrine of proportionality holds that treatments are ethically expendable when the benefits expected do not exceed the expected harms to the patient. While some people consider withholding of life-sustaining treatments morally more acceptable than withdrawing treatments that have begun, the dominant view today is that there is no morally significant difference between withholding and withdrawing. Thus, those who consider all behaviors that will result in death immoral will condemn both withholding and withdrawing (as well as active killing), and those that find withholding treatments on the grounds that there is not proportional benefit expected, likely consider withdrawing treatments acceptable on the same grounds. A treatment may be started because it is believed that expected benefits justify any necessary risks of harm. If, however, the treatment turns out not to offer the benefit originally expected, a patient or surrogate may withdraw the consent to the treatment leading to a justifiable withdrawal. These issues of deciding to accept or refuse treatment were explored in the cases of Chapter 8.

Many of the critical moral decisions related to the care of the terminally and critically ill actually involve the ethical issues of informed consent or refusal and withdrawal of consent. Both law and most ethical theories consider the moral principle of autonomy to take priority over paternalism. If this is true, then it is acceptable for the substantially autonomous patient to decline or withdraw consent, thus forgoing treatment even for life-sustaining situations.

There are some other problems related to care of the terminally ill patient that will be taken up in this chapter. These are problems that cannot be resolved solely by figuring out the relation among the duties to benefit the patient, respect autonomy, and avoid killing. The first section will focus on the problems of the definition of death. Then in succeeding sections the cases will deal with decisions by surrogates for terminally or critically ill patients who are not competent to make their own choices about care looking first at formerly competent patients, then at those who have never been competent. In the final section, the issue will be new controversies over limiting care to the terminally ill in order to conserve scarce medical resources.

THE DEFINITION OF DEATH

Until the late 1960s, there had been a millennium-old general understanding of what it meant to be dead. With the development of CPR, ventilators, and better understanding of pulmonary and cardiac physiology, we gained greater capacity to intervene in the dying process. We were able to uncouple a series of events that, until then, had always been connected. Now, for the first time, it was possible, thanks in part to respiratory care practitioners, to maintain cardiac and respiratory function even after brain function had been destroyed.

During this same period the first human heart transplant took place and society developed a profound interest in the viable organs that might be taken from dead patients. At this time we asked whether people could be considered dead if their heart and lung function continued but they had irreversibly lost the capacity for bodily integration. These patients have lost brain function known to be responsible for bodily integration. If such patients could be considered dead, then organs with life-saving potential could be procured. These developments gave rise to what is now thought of as the brain-oriented definition of death. According to it,

> An individual who has sustained either (1) irreversible cessation of circulatory and respiratory functions, or (2) irreversible cessation of all functions of the entire brain, including the brain stem, is dead. A determination of death must be made in accordance with accepted medical standards.[6]

Sometimes allied health professionals must confront cases that force them to determine exactly what it means for a patient to be dead. In this case we see that the now-fashionable definition based on irreversible loss of *all* brain function (the so-called "whole-brain-oriented" definition) is being challenged both by defenders of the more traditional "heart-and-lung-oriented" definition and by an even more revisionist "higher-brain-oriented" definition.

CASE 77: His Brain Is Gone But Is He Dead?

Wilber Harrison was deposited at an emergency room door about 11:30 P.M. by friends who departed quickly. He was a 34-year-old man whose appearance signaled a hard life on the streets of this major East Coast city. When the emergency room personnel found him he was not breathing and his heart was not beating. After emergency resuscitation, they stabilized the patient. Blood tests confirmed the suspicion of a heroin overdose.

He was moved on to the hospital floor, and after a week it became increasingly clear that while his heart continued to beat and lung function was maintained with a ventilator, he had suffered severe, permanent brain damage as a result of the respiratory depression undoubtedly caused by the heroin.

Mr. Harrison's family was located and informed of the bleak prognosis. Although the parents were Baptists, they acknowledged that Mr. Harrison had no religious affiliation. The neurologists confirmed a diagnosis of the destruction of the brain using the criteria of the Consultants to the President's Commission for the Study of Ethical Problems in Medicine and Biomedical and Behavioral Research.[7] The consulting neurologist reported that the patient was dead based on irreversible loss of brain function. The health care team could now proceed to discuss organ procurement with the family or, if organ procurement was not to be pursued, simply withdraw the ventilator as would normally be done on any deceased patient.

Molly Weinstein was horrified at what she heard. She was the respiratory care practitioner responsible for maintenance of Mr. Harrison's ventilatory support. She saw her patient as a living, breathing patient whose heart function was still strong. Admittedly, he would not "live" long were the ventilator stopped; Ms. Weinstein knew that. But many of Ms. Weinstein's patients were in that situation. Were they really going to tell her that she must stop life support and take his organs? His body functions continued; he was warm and pink; it was as if he were sleeping.

Ms. Weinstein, a practicing Jew, was firmly of the belief that Mr. Harrison was still alive. For centuries patients in this condition would have been considered alive. Although then they would have lacked the capacity to maintain the life, now that we have that capacity Ms. Weinstein felt she had a moral duty to continue ventilatory support. Moreover, she had seen the electroencephalogram (EEG) used by the neurologist to confirm his diagnosis of irreversible and complete loss of brain function. She was sure that she saw small movements in the EEG lines when the gains were turned to their maximum. She asked the EEG technician about them. Michael Morton, the EEG technician, said that often they get artifacts on EEG, but he acknowledged that these were not artifacts. They were small electron potentials really coming from the brain. He assured Ms. Weinstein that it was routine and that death was often pronounced in the presence of these very small signs of electrical activity in the brain.

Ms. Weinstein was deeply disturbed by this. As a Jew, she had the distinct impression that her tradition would not only consider such a patient alive, but that the treatment ought to continue until the patient dies. Can she insist that she continue ventilating the patient on the grounds that he was alive and that his life should be preserved?

Ms. Weinstein is right that, even though patients such as Mr. Harrison would legally be considered dead in virtually all jurisdictions of the world, some, including some members of the Jewish tradition, reject the judgment that society should treat patients like Mr. Harrison as if they were dead. It is important to realize that there is no technical neurological disagreement here. All involved agree that the brain will never again regain any of its normal bodily integrating functions.

Mr. Harrison is what is popularly referred to as "brain dead." That is a bad term because it could mean either that the brain is dead in a still-living person or that the person as a whole should be considered dead because the brain is dead and integrating capacity is lost (even though heart and pulmonary function can be maintained by skilled professionals like Ms. Weinstein). If this patient is considered dead for legal and social purposes, then many important events can take place: his wife, if he had one, would become a widow; his possessions could be dispersed according to the provisions of his will; his health insurance would stop funding his medical care; and his life insurance would pay to his beneficiary. If he is dead, then the organ procurement team can, with proper permission, take his organs, something that cannot be done while he is alive, even if his brain is dead.

The dispute between Ms. Weinstein and other members of the health care team is not one that can be resolved by any skill in diagnosis or other technical way. The issue is whether society should treat such patients as Mr. Harrison as dead or alive, knowing that some organ systems continue to function even though the brain is gone. If society wants to consider persons alive who retain the capacity to respire and maintain circulation, Mr. Harrison is alive. If it wants to focus on the bodily integration capacities localized in the brain, he is dead.

The state of New Jersey has recently made a modification in its law defining death.[8] Realizing that the choice of a definition is a social rather than a technical matter, it was concerned about citizens such as Ms. Weinstein who reach philosophical or religious conclusions that patients such as Mr. Harrison should be considered alive.[9] That law states that, if persons have religious objections to a brain-oriented definition of death, they may execute an advance declaration stating that if they are ever in Mr. Harrison's condition, they should have their death pronounced on the basis of cardiac function loss. Mr. Harrison, being of no known religious persuasion, would not have this right since, even if he favored a heart-based definition of death, it would not be on religious grounds. Moreover, the law does not address the problem of a member of the health care team who might object to brain-oriented definitions as Ms. Weinstein does. Even if she were in New Jersey, she would not have the right to continue Mr. Harrison's ventilator.

Which definition of death is the right one? What can be done to protect Ms. Weinstein's rights if the law and the other members of the health care team support a brain-oriented definition?

The exchange between Ms. Weinstein and Mr. Morton, the EEG technician, raises still another issue. Mr. Morton correctly states that it is common practice to pronounce death even though small electrical potentials can still be seen on an EEG. Major documents on the measurement of death of the brain acknowledge this practice.[10] This is generally explained by claiming that these signs of small amounts of electrical activity reflect only cellular activity, not bodily integrating functions at the supercellular level.

Still these are signs that the brain is not totally dead and that functions persist (even if they are at the cellular or local level). Thus, patients with these signs of brain activity do not literally have dead brains; they do not fully meet the definition of death based on irreversible loss of *all* functions of the *entire* brain. Some critics are suggesting that the definition of death based on the functions of the whole brain may have to be changed once again, replacing it with what is often called a "higher" brain definition. According to it, a person will be considered dead for legal and social purposes when there is irreversible loss of higher function, often equated with consciousness, even if cellular level or functions of the lower part of the brain remain in place. Since the brain stem provides not only reflex reactions but controls respiration, some patients, including those in a persistent vegetative state, could be considered dead even though they continue to breathe on their own. Ms. Weinstein thus faces a choice among three major types of definitions of death: heart-lung, whole-brain, and higher-brain definitions. Which one should be used in Mr. Harrison's case, and what should Ms. Weinstein do if she disagrees with the one chosen?

FORMERLY COMPETENT PATIENTS

The cases of Chapters 5 and 13 address the ethical principle of autonomy and informed consent, which is usually seen as protecting autonomy. Those of Chapter 8 address the ethics of killing and letting patients die. Those cases examined whether refusals of life-sustaining efforts are ethical and, if so, under what circumstances. Most commentators now generally agree that if a mentally competent individual wants to refuse medical treatment, he or she has the legal and perhaps also the moral right to do so.

To attempt to avoid certain unwanted treatments, some people are now writing advance directives specifying which treatments they want and which ones they want to refuse.[11] Federal law requires that all patients, upon admission to a hospital, be offered an opportunity to discuss advance directives.[12]

If the patient remains conscious and competent to confirm the advance directive at the time of crisis, normally the patient's wishes will be followed, but most critically ill patients are so ill that they lapse into incompetence. Health providers worry that the patient's wishes may not be adequately clear or that the patient may have changed his or her mind. The following case illustrates the problem.

CASE 78: Whether to Override a Living Will

Katherine Meeks has recently been transferred from her position as a technologist in the chemistry laboratory of Holy Name Hospital to a generalist laboratory position in the wholly owned nursing home subsidiary of the hospital. She is very pleased with this move as it allows her much greater flexibility, gives her greater professional responsibility, and provides more opportunity to interact with the patients. The home is a skilled nursing facility with four units organized around the level of care needs of the patients.

Residents of the home are housed in the unit that provides them the most independence yet meets their needs for fundamental assistance, nursing, and medical care. As necessary, patients are moved from one unit to another to meet their health care needs.

Ms. Josephine Duncan has been a resident of the home since its establishment eight years earlier. She has been in good health with an amazing amount of agility for an 83-year-old. She has been living in the unit providing the lowest level of care. Ms. Meeks has taken to visiting Mrs. Duncan whenever she has work on the unit and has grown quite fond of the woman.

Ms. Meeks has learned all about Mrs. Duncan's family, her professional career as a piano player, her likes and dislikes, and her thoughts about death. Ms. Meeks knows that Mrs. Duncan has signed a living will donating all her functioning organs for transplantation and requesting "no prolonged medical treatment" in the event of her illness. She has stated repeatedly that she refuses to allow her life to be artificially prolonged when there is no hope of full recovery. She has led a full and rewarding life and wishes it to end with dignity.

Upon returning from her daily walk, Mrs. Duncan falls on the steps of the home and breaks her hip. She is taken to Holy Name Hospital where the fracture is set, then returned to the nursing home after three days. She is placed in the nursing unit providing the highest level of help as she is totally dependent upon others for everything.

When Ms. Meeks visits Mrs. Duncan she was surprised to see how ill she appears after only four days. Mrs. Duncan does not respond in her usual manner and is not as alert as normal. Over the next several days, Mrs. Duncan drifts in and out of consciousness and becomes semicomatose two weeks after the fall.

Ms. Meeks is called by the medical staff to participate in a cutdown on Mrs. Duncan so that blood samples can be obtained and an IV started. There is discussion of hyperalimentation to ensure an adequate protein intake. It is Ms. Meeks' belief that these procedures violate the wishes of the patient and negate her living will. Knowing Mrs. Duncan's wishes can she participate in this process?

This appears to be a case in which a patient has executed a valid advance directive indicating her desire not to have prolonged life-sustaining treatment. What possible reasons could the medical staff give to defend a judgment to override the directive?

One problem is that apparently her advance directive was rather vague. It asked for "no prolonged medical treatment." Should Ms. Meeks have objected at the first treatment after the fall? Should all treatment after she lapses into unconsciousness be omitted? Would that not foreclose the possibility that her condition could be temporary? Assuming Ms. Meeks remains convinced that Mrs. Duncan would not want the treatment, exactly which treatment is she refusing: the cut down, the blood samples, the IV, the hyperalimentation?

Another problem is that clinicians often fear that the patient might have changed her mind after writing the directive. If the patient remains conscious and competent, the judgment can be reaffirmed, but not in a case like this. Does the possibility that Mrs. Duncan may have changed her mind justify overriding her wishes?

Some scholars have recently argued that while autonomy requires honoring a patient's expressed refusal as long as she remains aware of her past views, some patients, including permanently unconscious patients such as Mrs. Duncan might be, have so lost contact with their former views that they are, in effect, different persons.[13] As such it makes no sense to respect the autonomy of the former person, when a "new person" now exists who may have different interests. If the new Mrs. Duncan's interests are served by the treatment, why should Ms. Meeks be bound by the wishes of the former individual?

The underlying moral issue is whether the principle of autonomy should continue to be relevant when the patient is no longer autonomous. One approach is to apply what can be called the principle of "autonomy-extended." It holds that an autonomous person's wishes remain governing unless there is evidence that the patient changed her mind while still autonomous. Is that the appropriate approach here?

If Ms. Meeks finds none of the arguments convincing justifications for continuing the treatment in apparent violation of Mrs. Duncan's advance directive, she may find herself confronting a situation in which she is asked to participate in a treatment for which she believes there is not an adequate informed consent. The *Code of Ethics* of the American branch of her professional organization, the American Society for Medical Technology, does not specifically address this kind of a case. It offers some general guidelines that would often seem correct, but may have unexpected implications in this case. It first commits its members to "safeguard the patient from incompetent or illegal practice by others."[14] It also says that "clinical laboratory professionals comply with relevant laws and regulations." These provisions might be interpreted as generating a requirement for Ms. Meeks to speak up for her patient, especially if she views the treatment without consent as an illegal act, which it probably is. But in the section dealing with relations with colleagues, the code emphasizes the duty to "actively strive to establish cooperative and insightful working relationships with other health professionals."[15] It seems certain that Ms. Meeks will appear to be challenging the notion of being a cooperative team player if she speaks up for her patient. Could the code be interpreted as authorizing or even requiring the sacrifice of the patient to promote cooperative relations with other members of the health care team? Finally, one who subscribes to the code acknowledges that he or she will "safeguard the dignity and privacy of patients."

If the physician in charge insists on proceeding with the cut down, what options are available for her? She could appeal to the hospital's ethics committee. That body might persuade the physician to change course, but what if it does not? Consider the following options: complaining to her supervisor, the hospital attorney, or the chief of medicine; withdrawing from the case in protest; or speaking with the patient's family. Are there other options for her?

In the previous case one possibility was that the allied health professional who believed that a patient was receiving treatment in violation of her advance directive might report the problem to the patient's family. In other cases it is the family that wants the advance directive overturned. Consider the following situation:

CASE 79: May Family Override an Advance Directive?

Daniel Jenkins is a 65-year-old male who had undergone triple bypass surgery. Five years after his surgery, Mr. Jenkins indicated to his physician that he did not want a lot of further heroics.

Mr. Jenkins has once again been hospitalized. It appears that his repairs are beginning to fail. After an apparent stroke, he slips into a coma. His family is consulted immediately. They inform the physician that they want Mr. Jenkins ventilated.

In reading the patient's chart before applying the ventilation, Olive Cannon, a respiratory care practitioner, sees that Mr. Jenkins had indicated that he did not want "any heroics." She contacts the physician who confirms that Mr. Jenkins had requested that no heroics, for example, ventilation, be applied. The physician, however, says that he is going to be guided by the family rather than the wishes of someone who is no longer competent and cannot complain. Ms. Cannon is in a quandary as to what to do now.

This case raises issues similar to those in the previous case except that here it is the family pressing for overturning the expressed wishes of the patient. What is the reason why the family is pressing for continued treatment? Is it for their welfare or the patient's? What difference does it make morally? There may well be good reasons legally and psychologically why the health care team might want to honor the family's wishes. They are more likely to create legal trouble than the patient. But are there moral reasons?

Assume that the patient's wishes are clear but the family nevertheless believes it is pursuing the patient's interest by seeking to overturn his advance directive. Is there some reason to believe that the family would know the patient's interests better than the patient himself does? Perhaps he is not refusing further treatment he calls heroic for his own interests. He may be doing so to serve his family's interests, such as sparing them the expense or burden of further care. If so, do they have the right to override him?

If the family has the capacity to judge his interests, the case may pose the classic conflict between patient welfare and patient autonomy. If autonomy can be extended into the period of incompetency, as was suggested in the previous case, does it always take precedence over the family's judgment? Is there any moral reason why the family should prevail?

NEVER COMPETENT PATIENTS

The previous cases involved patients who were once mentally competent who had formulated a view about their terminal care. They had written advance directives. The issue was whether physicians, family, or others had the right to override the directive. Many patients have never been sufficiently autonomous to formulate a plan about their terminal care. They are children, significantly retarded adults, or otherwise incapacitated people. Other patients were once competent and could have formulated their plans, but they have left no available evidence that they did. In such cases patient autonomy is an impossibility. Some other appeal is necessary. This is often expressed as the standard of patient *best interest*. Someone has to be designated as the surrogate for the patient, perhaps by court designation of a guardian.

Often, however, formal court proceedings are inappropriate either because there is not enough time or because there is an obvious surrogate available. For example, parents are the presumed decision makers for their children's health care, including terminal care. There is increasingly agreement that even if the next of kin is not legally designated as a surrogate, he or she is normally the appropriate surrogate.[16] Sometimes problems arise when surrogates make unexpected decisions. The following case illustrates the problems that can arise.

CASE 80: Parental Refusal of Life-and-Death Chemotherapy

Timmy Brown was an active 2-year-old boy living with his parents on an organic farm in rural Utah when he developed leukemia. His parents were deeply committed to the natural foods movement. They believed that chemicals were the source of many of the health problems of the world and were, hence, committed to growing their own food using natural, organic methods.

They were very upset when the local oncologist, Dr. Jim Sampson, told them that their son, Timmy, was seriously ill. They were more upset when he recommended that they be transferred to the university teaching hospital in a neighboring state where he could get the latest chemotherapy, which the physician believed would be their best chance of saving the boy's life. He said that even with the aggressive chemotherapy, Timmy only had a 50-50 chance of surviving more than a year.

Mr. and Mrs. Brown knew of the terrible side effects of chemotherapy and did not want to inflict that on their boy. They believed their more natural methods would work better and would spare him the trauma of traveling to another state and receiving what they viewed as toxic poison. They wanted to give Timmy macrobiotic rice and laetrile, which they believed, based on reports they had read in their natural foods newsletter, would cure the leukemia.

When Dr. Sampson realized their objection and recognized that they felt very strongly about using the natural healing method, he considered making a deal with them. He would consider trying to obtain chemically uncontaminated batches of laetrile if Mr. and Mrs. Brown would permit him to administer chemotherapy at the same time. He was convinced that the laetrile and rice would provide no benefit, but considered them reasonably innocuous. He was afraid that if he insisted that they go to the university oncology program, they would simply set out on their own to obtain the laetrile.

If Dr. Sampson were to make this deal, he decided he needed help from Jenny Chang, the chief dietitian at the local hospital where Dr. Sampson had privileges. He would need her to assess whether Timmy's nutrition would be adequate for a child suffering from leukemia if he continued to eat the rice diet and laetrile.

Ms. Chang was at first shocked with the proposal. She considered it beneath her professional dignity to be part of the arrangement involving dietary treatment of leukemia with what she considered to be nothing more than an unproven health food fad. She was convinced that neither the rice nor the laetrile would help. Before she could participate in designing a diet that incorporated the macrobiotic rice and laetrile, she needed to assess the proposal in light of her health professional duty to do what will benefit the patient. She thought that even if the adult had the right to use unproven remedies, they did not have the right to impose them on a child. Should she accept Dr. Sampson's request for help in designing the special diet?

Ms. Chang is about to make a decision in which the life of a small child may hang in the balance. If there is any autonomy at stake here, it surely is not that of the child. Is there any reason why the parents should have the autonomy to choose less than the best course for their child?

The moral and legal standard that is usually put forward for situations like this is the "best interest" standard: choosing the course that will be expected to be best for the incompetent patient. Both Dr. Sampson and Ms. Chang believed that transfer to the university hospital for the chemotherapy protocol would be best for Timmy. Is there any reason why they should yield to the Browns?

If the clinician is dealing with a patient whose wishes cannot be known and who has no relatives available, the traditional rule is to do what is possible to prolong life, at least until there has been a careful and deliberate decision, preferably with the help of some formal due process such as a court review, to forgo further treatment on the grounds it is doing no good. In cases in which patients have family members or other surrogates standing by, however, the decision-making structure may be much more complex.

It is well established that even if autonomous patients have the right to make strange treatment refusal choices in medicine, they do not have an unlimited right to do so for their children.[17] Jehovah's Witness parents, for example, do not have the right to refuse life-saving blood transfusions for their children, even if they are sincere in their belief that it is best for them and even if they have the right to refuse blood themselves.[18] Health professionals cannot force treatment against the parents' wishes on their own, but, using legal due process, they can obtain a court order temporarily taking custody of the child from the parent for purposes of authorizing the life-saving medical treatment.

At the same time society may not want to insist on surrogates doing the absolute best. Determining exactly what is best would be a difficult task and enforcement of such a requirement would demand constant vigilance and state intrusion on family life. Generally, in matters of family life—such as education choices and discipline—parents are given discretion.

Still there is a limit beyond which surrogates cannot go when acting for their wards. They cannot choose corporal punishment beyond limits. They cannot choose unapproved schools by uncertified teachers. We can call the standard the *limits of reasonableness.* Surrogates such as parents, according to this standard, would be obliged to try to do what they think is best. If they were within reason, health professionals would try to cooperate in the parents' treatment plan even if they were not convinced it was the best.

The codes of ethics of the various health professions generally have not incorporated this notion of giving surrogates a reasonable range of discretion in making health care decisions for their wards. If they address the matter at all, they speak vaguely of "doing what is best for the patient." They really have not contemplated the possibility that a parent may make a somewhat unusual request that, arguably, is still within the range of the reasonable.

The American Dietetic Association, for instance, has nothing specific to say about Ms. Chang's dilemma. It speaks vaguely of practicing according to "scientific principles and current information," which might seem to support Ms. Chang's resistance to the proposed use of laetrile and macrobiotic diet, but it also speaks of working "with respect for the unique needs and values of individuals."[19] It is not at all clear, however, that the writers of that phrase had in mind respecting parental values if it significantly jeopardized the welfare of their child.

Dr. Sampson and Ms. Chang might refuse to cooperate with Mr. and Mrs. Brown were they to insist on trying to get laetrile and macrobiotic rice alone. They might even seek a court order for the chemotherapy.

The plan being considered, however, is more complicated. It involves administering the alternative therapy along with the orthodox therapy. Should Ms. Chang cooperate in the proposed deal?

LIMITS BASED ON INTERESTS OF OTHERS

All the cases in this chapter examined thus far work in what can be called a "patient-centered" framework. They focus on patient benefit or patient autonomy. Either way the goal is to center on the patient. We saw, however, in Chapters 3 and 4 that some of the most important ethical conflicts today involve tensions between the patient and others in the society. The principle of social beneficence that underlies utilitarian reasoning holds that actions tend toward being right when they produce the most good overall considering both the good for the patient and others.

That is a controversial notion, often rejected in health care ethics in favor of a more exclusive focus on the welfare of the patient. But in Chapter 4 we saw that there is another way that the interests of others can enter the picture. The principle of justice holds that actions tend toward being right if they distribute goods to those who have special claims. Egalitarian justice, which dominates modern nonutilitarian thinking about justice, usually interprets this to mean distributing health care on the basis of need.

Since terminally ill patients would normally be thought of as being in great need, they might, according to egalitarian interpretations of justice, have claims to resources that cannot be sustained solely on the more utilitarian notion of maximizing total benefit to the society.

Terminally ill patients often require extremely expensive treatments, and those treatments often do not have much chance of producing substantial benefits. If we calculate expected benefit by multiplying the possible benefit times the probability of that benefit, the expected benefit can be very small. Hence, increasingly, there are controversies over the ethics of allocating expensive treatments to the terminally ill. The last case in this volume introduces what may be one of the most critical issues of health care ethics of the future.

CASE 81: Limiting Terminal Care to Benefit Others

Juanita Young is a respiratory care practitioner who works at White Cross Hospital. Her normal patient load is to care for six patients during her shift. One of her six patients is in a permanent vegetative state as a result of an automobile accident that occurred two years ago. This patient, Evelyn Hodges, is in a coma, but continues to have secretions, which require respiratory therapy twice per day. She has no family and no one at the hospital knows very much about her.

On Friday, three of Ms. Young's colleagues fail to report to work. Their patient loads are distributed to Ms. Young and four other respiratory care practitioners. Instead of six patients, Ms. Young now has nine to treat. The additional patients that she receives include two with cystic fibrosis and one with pneumonia. With her own six patients it soon becomes evident that Ms. Young is not going to be able to provide complete therapy for her entire patient load.

All the patients, except for Evelyn Hodges, are in reasonably good condition. Furthermore, there is tangible evidence that the other eight patients benefit from the respiratory therapy. Ms. Young's question is: If she has to cut back a little somewhere, is it not best to do so with Ms. Hodges?

Clearly, if Ms. Young has the time, she would continue to provide respiratory care for all nine of her patients or make sure more therapists are on duty. The fact, however, is that, at least in the short run, there is not much Ms. Young can do to increase the number of respiratory care practitioners and she cannot provide full, standard care. She will have to care for the nine, in one way or another.

As we saw in Chapter 4, there are two ways to approach the problem of allocating scarce resources. In this case, the resource that is scarce is Ms. Young's services. When she implies that the best course would be to cut back on the care Ms. Hodges would receive, she is probably using utilitarian reasoning. She is probably looking at the greatest good considering the total good adding up the good she would do for each patient. She would have to acknowledge that there is some risk to Ms. Hodges in doing that. Ms. Hodges' life might even be threatened. But Ms. Young may be willing to tolerate that risk. In fact, she may not believe continuing treatment actually serves her patient in any way. In the previous case we suggested that, for patients whose wishes about terminal care are not known and who do not have family available to serve as surrogate, it is wise to proceed conservatively, presuming that the patient's interest dictates treatment. That at least leads to errors on the side of life.

But even if Ms. Young presumes continued aggressive suctioning is in Ms. Hodges' interest, the treatment may still not be considered to be a great benefit to her. She is in a coma. She cannot suffer discomfort from lack of suctioning. Many would argue that even death might not be inappropriate at this point.

Ms. Young apparently concludes that if her goal is to maximize the sum total of the benefit for all her patients, then it would be "best" to cut back on Ms. Hodges.

But the principle of justice provides another perspective. Justice, in its egalitarian interpretation, requires identifying who is worst off and doing what is possible to benefit that person. It seems plausible that Ms. Hodges is among the worst off. That could mean that she has special claims to Ms. Young's time even if she will not benefit greatly.

One way out of this conflict would be to conclude that patients in a permanent vegetative state get no benefit at all from suctioning. Even if health providers have a duty to benefit the worst off, they are surely not required to provide care that provides no benefit at all. The hospital or insurer might seek agreement in advance that patients in a permanent vegetative state would not benefit by treatment beyond a reasonable time to confirm diagnosis. Would that justify limiting care at this point? If it would, would it also justify limiting care even if resources were not scarce?

Since there is no reason to believe that the hospital or insurer had sought agreement on such a policy and Ms. Hodges is among the worst off, does Ms. Young have a moral duty based in justice or fairness to give Ms. Hodges equal or priority treatment?

ENDNOTES

1. Paul Ramsey, *The Patient as Person* (New Haven, CT: Yale University Press, 1970).
2. Tom Beauchamp and Seymour Perlin, *Ethical Issues in Death and Dying* (Englewood Cliffs, NJ: Prentice Hall, 1978); Robert F. Weir, ed., *Ethical Issues in Death and Dying* (New York: Columbia University Press, 1977); Dennis J. Horan and David Mall, eds., *Death, Dying, and Euthanasia* (Washington, D.C.: University Publications of America, 1977); Robert F. Weir, ed., *Ethical Issues in Death and Dying*, 2nd ed. (New York: Columbia University Press, 1986); The Hastings Center, *Guidelines on the Termination of Life-Sustaining Treatment and the Care of the Dying* (Briarcliff Manor, NY: The Center, 1987); Cynthia Cohen, ed., *Casebook on the Termination of Life-Sustaining Treatment and the Care of the Dying* (Bloomington: Indiana University Press, 1988); Robert M. Veatch, *Death, Dying, and the Biological Revolution*, rev. ed. (New Haven, CT: Yale University Press, 1989).
3. J. David Bleich, "The Obligation to Heal in the Judaic Tradition: A Comparative Analysis," *Jewish Bioethics*, ed. Fred Rosner and J. David Bleich (New York: Sanhedrin Press, 1979), pp. 1-44.

4. American Medical Association, *Current Opinions of the Council on Ethical and Judicial Affairs of the American Medical Association: Including the Principles of Medical Ethics and Rules of the Council on Ethical and Judicial Affairs* (Chicago: AMA, 1989).
5. President's Commission for the Study of Ethical Problems in Medicine and Biomedical and Behavioral Research, *Deciding to Forego [sic] Life-Sustaining Treatment: Ethical, Medical, and Legal Issues in Treatment Decisions* (Washington, D.C.: U.S. Government Printing Office, 1983).
6. President's Commission for the Study of Ethical Problems in Medicine and Biomedical and Behavioral Research. *Defining Death: Medical, Legal and Ethical Issues in the Definition of Death* (Washington, D.C.: U.S. Government Printing Office, 1981), p. 2.
7. President's Commission for the Study of Ethical Problems in Medicine and Biomedical and Behavioral Research, "Report of the Medical Consultants on the Diagnosis of Death to the President's Commission for the Study of Ethical Problems in Medicine and Biomedical and Behavioral Research," in *Defining Death*, pp. 159-166.
8. New Jersey Declaration of Death Act (1991), *New Jersey Statutes Annotated*, Title 26, 6A-1 to 6A-8.
9. Robert S. Olick, "Brain Death, Religious Freedom, and Public Policy," *Kennedy Institute of Ethics Journal*, Vol. 1 (December 1991), pp. 275-288.
10. A. Earl Walker et al., "An Appraisal of the Criteria of Cerebral Death—A Summary Statement," *Journal of the American Medical Association*, Vol. 237 (1977), pp. 982-986.
11. For a sample of an advance directive, see Norman L. Cantor, "My Annotated Living Will," *Law, Medicine & Health Care*, Vol. 18 (Spring-Summer 1990), pp. 114-122; Sissela Bok, "Personal Directions for Care at the End of Life," *The New England Journal of Medicine*, Vol. 295 (1976), pp. 367-369; The Catholic Hospital Association, *Christian Affirmation of Life* (St. Louis: The Catholic Hospital Association, 1982); Concern for Dying. "A Living Will," n.d.; and Robert M. Veatch, *Death, Dying, and the Biological Revolution*, rev. ed., pp. 154-155. For discussions of the ethics of advanced directives, see Arthur J. Dyck, "Living Wills and Mercy Killing: An Ethical Assessment," *Bioethics and Human Rights: A Reader for Health Professionals*, eds. Bertram and Elsie Bandman (Boston: Little, Brown, 1978), pp. 132-138; Allen Buchanan, "Advance Directives and Personal Identity Problem," *Philosophy and Public Affairs*, Vol. 17, no. 4 (Fall 1988), pp. 277-302; and Allen E. Buchanan and Dan W. Brock, *Deciding for Others: The Ethics of Surrogate Decision Making* (Cambridge: Cambridge University Press, 1989).
12. Elizabeth Leibold McCloskey, "The Patient Self-determination Act," *Kennedy Institute of Ethics Journal*, Vol. 1 (June 1991), pp. 163-169.
13. Rebecca S. Dresser and John A. Robertson, "Quality of Life and Non-Treatment Decisions for Incompetent Patients: A Critique of the Orthodox Approach," *Law, Medicine, & Health Care*, Vol. 17 (1980), pp. 234-244; Buchanan and Brock, *Deciding for Others: The Ethics of Surrogate Decision Making*.

14. American Society for Medical Technology, *Code of Ethics* (Washington, D.C.: ASMT, n.d.).
15. Ibid.
16. Judith Areen, "The Legal Status of Consent Obtained from Families of Adult Patients to Withhold or Withdraw Treatment," *Journal of the American Medical Association*, Vol. 258, no. 2 (July 10, 1987), pp. 229-235; Robert M. Veatch, "Limits of Guardian Treatment Refusal: A Reasonableness Standard," *American Journal of Law and Medicine*, Vol. 9, no. 4 (Winter 1984), pp. 427-468.
17. Yolanda V. Vorys, "The Outer Limits of Parental Autonomy: Withholding Medical Treatment from Children," *Ohio State Law Journal*, Vol. 43, no. 3 (1981), pp. 813-829; President's Commission for the Study of Ethical Problems in Medicine and Biomedical and Behavioral Research, *Deciding to Forego [sic] Life-Sustaining Treatment*.
18. Maureen L. Moore, "Their Life Is in the Blood: Jehovah's Witnesses, Blood Transfusions and the Courts," *Northern Kentucky Law Review*, Vol. 10, no. 2 (1983), pp. 281-304.
19. The American Dietetic Association, *Code of Ethics for the Profession of Dietetics and Review Process for Alleged Violations* (Chicago: ADA, 1991).

INDIVIDUAL CONTRIBUTORS TO CASE STUDIES

Professor Carole C. Burnette
Department of Physical Therapy
Howard University
Washington, DC

Patricia A. Bynum
Nuclear Medicine Technologist
Sibley Memorial Hospital
Washington, DC

Ruth A. Hansen, Ph.D., OTR, FAOTA
Professor, Eastern Michigan University
Ypsilanti, MI

Elizabeth M. Kanny, MA, OTRL/L, FAOTA
Head, Division of Occupational Therapy
Department of Rehabilitation Medicine
University of Washington
Seattle, WA

Penny Kyler-Hutchison, MA, OTR/L, FAOTA
Ethics Program Manager
Professional Development Division
The American Occupational Therapy Association, Inc.
Bethesda, MD

Lisa W. Mitchell, MAS, RD, LD
Food Service Director
Food and Nutrition Services
Marriott Corporation at Loudoun Hospital Center
Leesburg, VA

Professor Elaine O. Patrikas
Department of Health Information Management
Temple University
Philadelphia, PA

Dr. Glenda D. Price
Provost
Spelman College
Atlanta, GA

Dr. Mattie J. Tabron
Associate Professor and Director,
Radiation Therapy Department
Howard University Hospital
Washington, DC

Professor Peggy Valentine
Department of Community Health and Family Practice
Howard University
Washington, DC

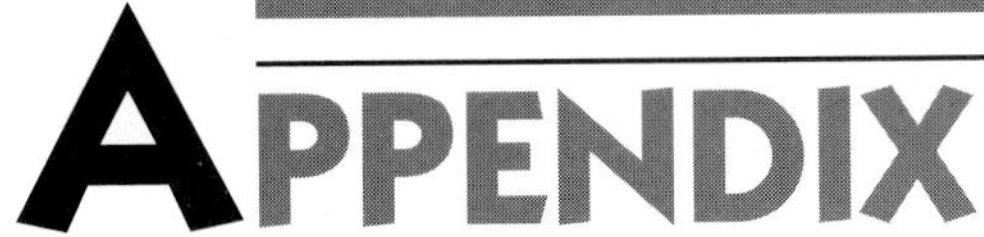

Appendix

Allied Health Codes of Ethics

The American Dietetics Association Code of Ethics for the Profession of Dietetics ©1993. Used by permission.

Introduction

The American Dietetic Association and its Commission on Dietetic Registration are in the vanguard of professional associations and credentialing bodies that have adopted a voluntary, enforceable code of ethics. This code, entitled the *Code of Ethics for the Profession of Dietetics*, challenges all members, registered dietitians, and dietetic technicians, registered, to uphold ethical principles. The enforcement process for the Code of Ethics, which took effect on January 1, 1989, establishes a fair system to deal with complaints about members and credentialed practitioners from peers or the public.

The first code of ethics in the professions was adopted by the American Medical Association in 1848. Since that time, many other professional societies have established codes to protect consumers and other professionals from improper conduct.

The Standards of Professional Responsibility, the predecessor of the current Code, were adopted by the House of Delegates in October 1982, with enforcement beginning in 1985. The current *Code of Ethics for the Profession of Dietetics* was developed to apply to all members and credentialed practitioners. It was adopted by the House of Delegates in October 1987.

The Ethics Committee of the Board of Directors is responsible for reviewing, promoting, and enforcing the Code. The Committee also educates members, credentialed practitioners, students, and the public about the ethical principles contained in the Code. Support of the *Code of Ethics* by members and credentialed practitioners is vital to guiding the profession's actions and to strengthening its credibility.

Code of Ethics for the Profession of Dietetics

Preamble

The American Dietetic Association and its credentialing agency, the Commission on Dietetic Registration, believe it is in the best interests of the profession and the public it serves that a Code of Ethics provide guidance to dietetic practitioners in their professional practice and conduct. Dietetic practitioners have voluntarily developed a Code of Ethics to reflect the ethical principles guiding the dietetic profession and to outline commitments and obligations of the dietetic practitioner to self, client, society, and the profession.

The purpose of the Commission on Dietetic Registration is to assist in protecting the nutritional health, safety, and welfare of the public by establishing and enforcing qualifications for dietetic registration and for issuing voluntary credentials to individuals who have attained those qualifications. The Commission has adopted this Code to apply to individuals who hold these credentials.

The Ethics Code applies in its entirety to members of The American Dietetic Association who are registered dietitians (RDs) or dietetic technicians, registered (DTRs). Except for sections solely dealing with the credential, the Code applies to all ADA members who are not RDs or DTRs. Except for aspects solely dealing with membership, the Code applies to all RDs and DTRs who are not ADA members. All of the aforementioned are referred to in the Code as "dietetic practitioners."

Principles

1. The dietetic practitioner provides professional services with objectivity and with respect for the unique needs and values of individuals.
2. The dietetic practitioner avoids discrimination against other individuals on the basis of race, creed, religion, sex, age, and national origin.
3. The dietetic practitioner fulfills professional commitments in good faith.
4. The dietetic practitioner conducts him/herself with honesty, integrity, and fairness.
5. The dietetic practitioner remains free of conflict of interest while fulfilling the objectives and maintaining the integrity of the dietetic profession.
6. The dietetic practitioner maintains confidentiality of information.
7. The dietetic practitioner practices dietetics based on scientific principles and current information.
8. The dietetic practitioner assumes responsibility and accountability for personal competence in practice.
9. The dietetic practitioner recognizes and exercises professional judgment within the limits of his/her qualifications and seeks counsel or makes referrals as appropriate.
10. The dietetic practitioner provides sufficient information to enable clients to make their own informed decisions.
11. The dietetic practitioner who wishes to inform the public and colleagues of his/her services does so by using factual information. The dietetic practitioner does not advertise in a false or misleading manner.

12. The dietetic practitioner promotes or endorses products in a manner that is neither false nor misleading.
13. The dietetic practitioner permits use of his/her name for the purpose of certifying that dietetic services have been rendered only if he/she has provided or supervised the provision of those services.
14. The dietetic practitioner accurately presents professional qualifications and credentials.
    A. The dietetic practitioner uses "RD" or "registered dietitian" and "DTR" or "dietitian technician, registered," only when registration is current and authorized by the Commission on Dietetic Registration.
    B. The dietetic practitioner provides accurate information and complies with all requirements of the Commission on Dietetic Registration program in which he/she is seeking initial or continues credentials from the Commission on Dietetic Registration.
    C. The dietetic practitioner is subject to disciplinary action for aiding another person in violating any Commission on Dietetic Registration requirements or aiding another person in representing himself/herself as an RD or DTR when he/she is not.
15. The dietetic practitioner presents substantiated information and interprets controversial information without personal bias, recognizing that legitimate differences of opinion exist.
16. The dietetic practitioner makes all reasonable effort to avoid bias in any kind of professional evaluation. The dietetic practitioner provides objective evaluation of candidates for professional association membership, awards, scholarships, or job advancements.
17. The dietetic practitioner voluntarily withdraws from professional practice under the following circumstances:
    A. The dietetic practitioner has engaged in any substance abuse that could affect his/her practice.
    B. The dietetic practitioner has been adjudged by a court to be mentally incompetent.
    C. The dietetic practitioner has an emotional or mental disability that affects his/her practice in a manner that could harm the client.
18. The dietetic practitioner complies with all applicable laws and regulations concerning the profession. The dietetic practitioner is subject to disciplinary action under the following circumstances:
    A. The dietetic practitioner has been convicted of a crime under the laws of the United States which is a felony or a misdemeanor, an essential element of which is dishonesty, and which is related to the practice of the profession.

B. The dietetic practitioner has been disciplined by a state, and at least one of the grounds for the discipline is the same or substantially equivalent to these principles.

C. The dietetic practitioner has committed an act of misfeasance or malfeasance which is directly related to the practice of the profession as determined by a court of competent jurisdiction, a licensing board, or an agency of a governmental body.

19. The dietetic practitioner accepts the obligation to protect society and the profession by upholding the Code of Ethics for the Profession of Dietetics and by reporting alleged violations of the Code through the defined review process of The American Dietetic Association and its credentialing agency, the Commission on Dietetic Registration.

Review Process for Alleged Violations of the Code of Ethics for the Profession of Dietetics

Procedures for review process

1. Complaint. A complaint that a dietetic practitioner has allegedly violated the Code of Ethics for the Profession of Dietetics will be submitted in writing on the appropriate form to the Ethics Committee in care of the Executive Department of The American Dietetic Association.

The complaint must be made within one year of the date that the complainant (person making complaint) first became aware of the alleged violation or within one year from the issuance of a final decision in an administrative, licensure board, or judicial action involving the facts asserted in the complaint.

The complainant need not be a member of The American Dietetic Association or a practitioner credentialed by the Commission on Dietetic Registration.

The complaint must contain details on the activities complained of the basis for complainant's knowledge of these activities, names, addresses, and telephone numbers of all persons involved or who might have knowledge of the activities, and whether the complaint has been submitted to a court, administrative body, or a state licensure board. The complaint must also cite the section(s) of the Code of Ethics for the Profession of Dietetics allegedly violated.

The complaint must be signed and sworn to by the complainant(s).

2. Preliminary review of complaint. The chairman of the Ethics Committee, General Counsel of The American Dietetic Association, and appropriate staff will review the complaint to determine if all the required information has been submitted by the complainant and whether an ethics question is involved.

If a complaint is made regarding an alleged violation of the Code of Ethics for the Profession of Dietetics and a similar complaint is already under consideration regarding the same individual by a state licensure board of examiners, an administrative body or a court of law, the Ethics Committee will not process the complaint until a final decision has been issued.

3. Response. If the persons making this preliminary review determine that the process should proceed, the chairman of the Ethics Committee will notify the respondent (person against whom the complaint is made) that a complaint has been made.

The notice will be sent from the Executive Department via certified mail, return receipt requested. The respondent will be sent a copy of the complaint, the Code of Ethics for the Profession of Dietetics, the Review Process, and a Response to Complaint form.

The respondent will have thirty (30) days from receipt of the notification in which to submit a response. The response must be signed and sworn to by the respondent(s).

If the Ethics Committee does not receive a response, the chairman of the Ethics committee or his/her designee will contact the respondent by telephone. If contact with the respondent is still not made, a written notice will be sent. Failure to reach the respondent will not prevent the committee from proceeding with an investigation.

4. Disposition. If the Chairman of the Ethics Committee deems it appropriate after consultation with the General Counsel and appropriate staff, he/she will submit the complaint and the response to the Ethics Committee for review.

The committee will reach a decision as to the disposition of the complaint, either: (1) that the complaint and response, jointly, do not present an ethics issue; (2) that the issues(s) involved do not warrant a hearing; or (3) that the Ethics Committee conduct a hearing.

The Ethics Committee will notify the complainant and the respondent of the decision.

5. Remedial action. At any time prior to the hearing, the Ethics Committee chairman may recommend appropriate remedial action to the parties, which if agreed to by the respondent, would resolve the matter.

When the Ethics Committee is informed by a state licensure body that a person subject to the Code of Ethics for the Profession of Dietetics has had his/her license suspended or revoked for reasons covered by the Code, the Ethics Committee shall review the record and may take appropriate disciplinary action without a formal hearing.

6. Preparation for hearing. Hearing dates will be established by the chairman of the Ethics Committee. All hearings will be held in Chicago.

The Ethics Committee will notify the respondent and the complainant by certified mail, return receipt requested, of the date, time, and place of the hearing.

The respondent may request a copy of the file on the case and will be allowed at least one postponement, provided the request for postponement is received by The American Dietetic Association at least fourteen (14) days before the hearing date.

7. **Hearings.** The Chairman of the Ethics Committee will conduct a hearing with the General Counsel and appropriate staff present. The parties shall have the right to appear, to present witnesses and evidence; to cross-examine the opposing party and adverse witnesses; and to have legal counsel present. Legal counsel for the parties may advise their clients, but may only participate in the hearings with the permission of the chairman.

The hearing is the sole opportunity for the participants to present their position.

Three members of the Ethics Committee shall constitute a quorum. Affirmative vote of two-thirds (2/3) of the members voting will be required to reach a decision.

A transcript will be prepared and will be available to the parties at cost.

8. **Costs.** The American Dietetic Association will bear the costs for the hearing committee, the ADA General Counsel, ADA staff, and any other parties called by the ADA. The American Dietetic Association will bear the travel and one night's hotel expenses for the complainant and respondent and one person that each chooses to bring, provided that such person is necessary to the conduct of the hearing as determined by the Chairman of the Ethics Committee. The Ethics Committee shall issue regulations to govern the payment of these expenses which shall be incorporated and made part of these procedures.

The respondent and the complainant will be responsible for all costs and fees incurred in their preparation for and attendance at the hearing, except expenses for travel and hotel as stated above.

9. **Decision.** The Ethics Committee will render a written decision specifying the reasons therefor and citing the provision(s) of the Code of Ethics for the Profession of Dietetics that has/have been violated. The Committee will decide:

A. That the respondent be acquitted; or

B. That the respondent be censured, placed on probation, suspended, or expelled from The American Dietetic Association; and/or

C. That the credential of the respondent be suspended or revoked by the Commission on Dietetic Registration of The American Dietetic Association.

Censure—A written reprimand expressing disapproval of conduct. It carries no loss of membership or registration status, but may result in removal from office at the national, state, and district levels and from committee membership.
Time frame—not applicable.
Probation—A directive to allow for correction of behavior specified in Principle 17 of the Code of Ethics for the Profession of Dietetics. It may include mandatory participation in, remedial programs (e.g., education, professional counseling, peer assistance). Failure to successfully complete these programs may result in other disciplinary action being taken. It carries no loss of membership or registration status, but may result in removal from office at the national, state, and district levels and from committee membership.
Time frame—specified time to be decided on a case-by-case basis.
Suspension—Temporary loss of membership and all membership benefits and privileges for a specified time with the exception of retention of coverages under health and disability insurance. ADA group malpractice insurance will not be available and will not be renewed during the suspension period.
Time frame—specified time to be decided on a case-by-case basis.
Suspension of registration—Temporary loss of credential and all benefits and privileges for a specified period of time. It may include mandatory participation in remedial programs (e.g., education, professional counseling, peer assistance).
At the end of the specified suspension period, membership and registration benefits and privileges are automatically restored.
Time frame—specified time to be decided on a case-by-case basis.
Expulsion—Removal from membership and a loss of all benefits and privileges.
Time frame—may apply for reinstatement after a five- year period has elapsed or sooner if the basis for the expulsion has been removed, with payment of a reinstatement fee. Must meet membership requirements in effect at the time of application for reinstatement.
Revocation of credential—Loss of registration status and removal from registry; loss of all benefits and privileges. Upon revocation, the former credentialed practitioner shall return the registration identification card to the Commission on Dietetic Registration.
Time frame—Specified time for reapplication to be decided on a case-by-case basis. A credential will not be issued until the Commission on Dietetic Registration determines that the reasons for revocation have been removed.

The decision of the Ethics Committee will be sent to the respondent and the complainant as soon as practicable after the hearing.

10. Appeals. Only the respondent may appeal an adverse decision to The American Dietetic Association Appeals Committee.

During the appeals process, the membership and registration status of the respondent remain unchanged.

A. Recourse to the Appeals Committee. To request a hearing before the Appeals Committee, the respondent/appellant shall notify the appropriate staff at ADA headquarters, by certified mail, return receipt requested, that the respondent wishes to appeal the decision. This notification must be received within thirty (30) calendar days after receipt of the letter advising the respondent/appellant of the Ethics Committee's decision.

1) The appeal must be in writing and contain, at a minimum, the following information:
   a. The decision being appealed
   b. The date of the decision
   c. Why the individual feels the decision is wrong or was improperly rendered (See 10, B, (4), *Scope of review*, below)
   d. The redress sought by the individual.

The appeal will be signed and sworn to. If the appeal does not contain the information listed above, it will be returned to the individual who will be given ten (10) calendar days to resubmit. Failure to furnish the required information within ten (10) calendar days will result in the appeal being waived.

2) Upon receipt of this notification, appropriate staff shall promptly notify the chairman of the Appeals Committee that the respondent/appellant is appealing a decision made by the Ethics Committee.
3) The Appeals Committee chairman shall acknowledge the appeal and request a copy of the relevant written information on the case from appropriate staff.

B. Procedures for appeals.

1) Composition of Appeals Committee. The Appeals Committee shall consist of an Appeals Committee member serving as presiding officer, two members selected from the Appeals Panel, one technical advisor from the ADA headquarters staff, and ADA's General Counsel.
2) Participants at appeal hearings.
   a. All appeals hearings will be held in Chicago. The complainant/appellee, the respondent/appellant, and the chairman of the Ethics Committee will have the opportunity to participate in the appeals hearing.

b. The parties may have legal counsel present, who may advise their clients, but may only participate in the hearings with the permission of the chairman.
c. Attendance at the hearing will be limited to persons determined by the chairman to have a direct connection with the appeal.

3) Conduct of the hearing. The three parties involved in the appeal will be given the opportunity to state why the decision and/or disciplinary action of the Ethics Committee should be upheld, modified, or reversed.
4) Scope of review. The Appeals Committee will determine whether the Ethics Committee committed a procedural error that affected its decision, whether the Ethics Committee's decision was contrary to the weight of the evidence presented to it, or whether there is new and substantial evidence that would likely have affected the Ethics Committee's decision that was unavailable to the parties at the time of the Ethics Committee's hearing for reasons beyond their control.
In reviewing the Ethics Committee's decision, the Appeals Committee shall consider only the transcript of the hearing and the evidence presented to the Ethics Committee.
5) Record of hearing. A transcript will be prepared and will be maintained in the case file.
6) Decision of Appeals Committee.
a. The Appeals Committee shall prepare a written decision stating the reasons therefor. The decision shall be to affirm, modify, or reject the decision and/or disciplinary action of the Ethics Committee or to remand the case to the Ethics Committee with instructions for further proceedings.
b. Decisions of the Appeals Committee will be final.

C. Costs. The American Dietetic Association will bear the costs for the Appeals Committee, the ADA General Counsel, ADA staff, and any parties called by the ADA. The ADA will bear the travel and one night's hotel expenses for the respondent/appellant, the complainant/appellee, and the chairman of the Ethics Committee. The Ethics Committee shall issue regulations to govern the payment of these expenses which shall be incorporated and made part of this procedure.
The respondent/appellant and the complainant/appellee will be responsible for all costs and fees incurred in their preparation for and attendance at the hearing, except expenses for travel and hotel as stated above.

11. Notification of adverse action. If the respondent is disciplined by the Ethics Committee and does not appeal the decision, the chairman of the Ethics Committee will notify the appropriate American Dietetic Association organization units, CDR, the state dietetic association, appropriate licensure boards, and governmental and private bodies within thirty (30) days after notification of the final decision.

In the event the respondent appeals a decision to discipline him/her and the Ethics Committee decision is affirmed or modified, similar notification will be made by the chairman of the Ethics Committee.

Disclosure of disciplinary action by the Ethics Committee following final appeal will be published in the *Journal of The American Dietetic Association*, the *ADA Courier*, and other ADA publications approved by the Ethics Committee. A registered dietitian or dietetic technician, registered, whose credential has been suspended or revoked will have that fact noted if inquiries are made to the Office on Dietetic Credentialing at ADA headquarters.

12. Recordkeeping.

A. Records will be kept for a period of time after the disposition of the case in the Executive Department in accordance with ADA's record retention policy.

B. Information will be provided only upon written request and affirmative response from ADA's General Counsel.

Confidentiality Procedures

The following procedures have been developed to protect the confidentiality of both the complainant and the respondent in the investigation of a complaint of an alleged violation of the Code of Ethics for the Profession of Dietetics.

1. The need for confidentiality will be stressed in initial communications with all parties.
2. Committee members will refrain from discussing the complaint and hearing outside of official committee business pertaining to the complaint and hearing.
3. If the hearing on a complaint carries over to the next committee, the complaint will be heard by the original committee to consider the complaint.
4. Communication with ADA witnesses will be the responsibility of the committee chairman or staff liaison.
5. Witnesses who testify on behalf of ADA will be informed of the confidentiality requirements and agree to abide by them.
6. The committee chairman will stress the importance of confidentiality at the time of the hearing.

7. To ensure confidentiality, the only record of the hearing will be the official transcript and accompanying materials which will be kept at the ADA offices. All other materials that were mailed or distributed to committee members should be returned to ADA staff along with any notes taken by committee members.
8. The transcript will be available if there is an appeal of the Ethics Committee's decision only to the parties, Ethics Committee members, Appeals Committee members, and staff directly involved with the appeal.

American Health Information Management Association Code of Ethics Amended October 1991. Used with permission.

Preamble

The health information management professional abides by a set of ethical principles developed to safeguard the public and to contribute within the scope of the profession to quality and efficiency in health care. This Code of Ethics, adopted by the members of the American Health Information Management Association, defines the standards of behavior which promote ethical conduct.

Principles

1. The Health Information Management Professional demonstrates behavior that reflects integrity, supports objectivity, and fosters trust in professional activities.
2. The Health Information Management Professional respects the dignity of each human being.
3. The Health Information Management Professional strives to improve personal competence and quality of services.
4. The Health Information Management Professional represents truthfully and accurately professional credentials, education, and experience.
5. The Health Information Management Professional refuses to participate in illegal or unethical acts and also refuses to conceal the illegal, incompetent, or unethical acts of others.
6. The Health Information Management Professional protects the confidentiality of primary and secondary health records as mandated by law, professional standards, and the employer's policies.
7. The Health Information Management Professional promotes to others the tenets of confidentiality.

8. The Health Information Management Professional adheres to pertinent laws and regulations while advocating changes which serve the best interest of the public.
9. The Health Information Management Professional encourages appropriate use of health record information and advocates policies and systems that advance the management of health records and health information.
10. The Health Information Management Professional recognizes and supports the Association's mission.

American Society for Clinical Laboratory Sciences Code of Ethics of the American Society for Medical Technology June, 1995. Used with permission.

Preamble

The Code of Ethics of the American Society for Medical Technology (ASMT) sets forth the principles and standards by which clinical laboratory professionals practice their profession.

The professional conduct of clinical laboratory professionals is based on the following duties and principles:

I. Duty of the Patient

Clinical laboratory professionals are accountable for the quality and integrity of the laboratory services they provide. This obligation includes continuing competence in both judgment and performance as individual practitioners, as well as in striving to safeguard the patient from incompetent or illegal practice by others.

Clinical laboratory professionals maintain high standards of practice and promote the acceptance of such standards at every opportunity. They exercise sound judgment in establishing, performing and evaluating laboratory testing.

Clinical laboratory professionals perform their services with regard for the patient as an individual, respecting his or her right to confidentiality, the uniqueness of his or her needs and his or her right to timely access to needed services. Clinical laboratory professionals provide accurate information to others about the services they provide.

II. Duty to Colleagues and the Profession

Clinical laboratory professionals accept responsibility to individually contribute to the advancement of the profession through a variety of activities. These activities include contributions to the body of knowledge of the profession; establishing and implementing high standards of practice and education; seeking fair socioeconomic working conditions for themselves and other members of the profession, and holding their colleagues and the profession in high regard and esteem.

Clinical laboratory professionals actively strive to establish cooperative and insightful working relationships with other health professionals, keeping in mind their primary objective to ensure a high standard of care for the patients they serve.

III. Duty to Society

Clinical laboratory professionals share with other citizens the duties of responsible citizenship. As practitioners of an autonomous profession, they have the responsibility to contribute from their sphere of professional competence to the general well-being of the community, and specifically to the resolution of social issues affecting their practice and collective good.

Clinical laboratory professionals comply with relevant laws and regulations pertaining to the practice of clinical laboratory science and actively seek, within the dictates of their consciences, to change those which do not meet the high standards of care and practice to which the profession is committed.

As a clinical laboratory professional, I acknowledge my professional responsibility to:

Maintain and promote standards of excellence in performing and advancing the art and science of my profession;
Safeguard the dignity and privacy of patients;
Hold my colleagues and my profession in high esteem and regard;
Contribute to the general well-being of the community; and
Actively demonstrate my commitment to these responsibilities throughout my professional life.

The American Occupational Therapy Association, Inc.
Occupational Therapy Code of Ethics
© 1994. Reprinted with permission.

The American Occupational Therapy Association's Code of Ethics is a public statement of the values and principles used in promoting and maintaining high standards of behavior in occupational therapy. The American Occupational Therapy Association and its members are committed to furthering people's ability to function within their total environment. To this end, occupational therapy personnel provide services for individuals in any stage of health and illness, to institutions, to other professionals and colleagues, to students, and to the general public.

The Occupational Therapy Code of Ethics is a set of principles that applies to occupational therapy personnel at all levels. The roles of practitioner (registered occupational therapist and certified occupational therapy assistant), educator, fieldwork educator, supervisor, administrator, consultant, fieldwork coordinator, faculty program director, researcher/scholar, entrepreneur, student, support staff, and occupational therapy aide are assumed.

Any action that is in violation of the spirit and purpose of this Code shall be considered unethical. To ensure compliance with the Code, enforcement procedures are established and maintained by the Commission on Standards and Ethics. Acceptance of membership in the American Occupational Therapy Association commits members to adherence to the Code of Ethics and its enforcement procedures.

Principle 1.

Occupational therapy personnel shall demonstrate a concern for the well-being of the recipients of their services. (Beneficence)

A. Occupational therapy personnel shall provide services in an equitable manner for all individuals.
B. Occupational therapy personnel shall maintain relationships that do not exploit the recipient of services sexually, physically, emotionally, financially, socially or in any other manner. Occupational therapy personnel shall avoid those relationships or activities that interfere with professional judgment and objectivity.
C. Occupational therapy personnel shall take all reasonable precautions to avoid harm to the recipient of services or to his or her property.
D. Occupational therapy personnel shall strive to ensure that fees are fair, reasonable, and commensurate with the service performed and are set with due regard for the service recipient's ability to pay.

Principle 2.

Occupational therapy personnel shall respect the rights of the recipients of their services. (e.g., Autonomy, Privacy, Confidentiality)

A. Occupational therapy personnel shall collaborate with service recipients or their surrogate(s) in determining goals and priorities throughout the intervention process.
B. Occupational therapy personnel shall fully inform the service recipients of the nature, risks, and potential outcomes of any interventions.
C. Occupational therapy personnel shall obtain informed consent from subjects involved in research activities indicating they have been fully advised of the potential risks and outcomes.

D. Occupational therapy personnel shall respect the individual's right to refuse professional services or involvement in research or educational activities.
E. Occupational therapy personnel shall protect the confidential nature of information gained from educational, practice, research, and investigational activities.

Principle 3.

Occupational therapy personnel shall achieve and continually maintain high standards of competence. (Duties)

A. Occupational therapy practitioners shall hold the appropriate national and state credentials for providing services.
B. Occupational therapy personnel shall use procedures that conform to the Standards of Practice of the American Occupational Therapy Association.
C. Occupational therapy personnel shall take responsibility for maintaining competence by participating in professional development and educational activities.
D. Occupational therapy personnel shall perform their duties on the basis of accurate and current information.
E. Occupational therapy practitioners shall protect service recipients by ensuring that duties assumed by or assigned to other occupational therapy personnel are commensurate with their qualifications and experience.
F. Occupational therapy practitioners shall provide appropriate supervision to individuals for whom the practitioners have supervisory responsibility.
G. Occupational therapists shall refer recipients to other service providers or consult with other service providers when additional knowledge and expertise are required.

Principle 4.

Occupational therapy personnel shall comply with laws and Association polices guiding the profession of occupational therapy. (Justice)

A. Occupational therapy personnel shall understand and abide by applicable Association policies; local, state, and federal laws; and institutional rules.
B. Occupational therapy personnel shall inform employers, employees, and colleagues about those laws and Association policies that apply to the profession of occupational therapy.
C. Occupational therapy practitioners shall require those they supervise in occupational therapy related activities to adhere to the Code of Ethics.

D. Occupational therapy personnel shall accurately record and report all information related to professional activities.

Principle 5.

Occupational therapy personnel shall provide accurate information about occupational therapy services. (Veracity)

A. Occupational therapy personnel shall accurately represent their qualifications, education, experience, training, and competence.
B. Occupational therapy personnel shall disclose any affiliations that may pose a conflict of interest.
C. Occupational therapy personnel shall refrain from using or participating in the use of any form of communication that contains false, fraudulent, deceptive, or unfair statements or claims.

Principle 6.

Occupational therapy personnel shall treat colleagues and other professionals with fairness, discretion, and integrity. (Fidelity, Veracity)

A. Occupational therapy personnel shall safeguard confidential information about colleagues and staff.
B. Occupational therapy personnel shall accurately represent the qualifications, views, contributions, and findings of colleagues.
C. Occupational therapy personnel shall report any breaches of the Code of Ethics to the appropriate authority.

American Academy of Physician Assistants Guidelines for Professional Conduct March 1992. Used with permission.

The American Academy of Physician Assistants recognizes its responsibility to aid the profession in maintaining high standards in the provision of quality and accessible health care services. The following principles delineate the standards governing the conduct of physician assistants in their professional interactions with patients, colleagues, other health professionals and the general public. Realizing that no code can encompass all ethical responsibilities of the physician assistant, this enumeration of obligations in the Code of Ethics is not comprehensive and does not constitute a denial of the existence of other obligations, equally imperative, though not specifically mentioned.

Physician assistants shall be committed to providing competent medical care, assuming as their primary responsibility the health, safety, welfare and dignity of all humans.

Physician assistants shall extend to each patient the full measure of their ability as dedicated, empathetic health care providers and shall assume responsibility for the skillful and proficient transactions of their professional duties.

Physician assistants shall deliver needed health care services to health consumers without regard to sex, age, race, creed, socioeconomic and political status.

Physician assistants shall adhere to all state and federal laws governing informed consent concerning the patient's health care.

Physician assistants shall seek consultation with their supervising physician, other health providers, or qualified professionals having special skills, knowledge or experience whenever the welfare of the patient will be safeguarded or advanced by such consultation. Supervision should include ongoing communication between the physician and the physician assistant regarding the care of all patients.

Physician assistants shall take personal responsibility for being familiar with and adhering to all federal/state laws applicable to the practice of their profession.

Physician assistants shall provide only those services for which they are qualified via education and/or experience and by pertinent legal regulatory process.

Physician assistants shall not misrepresent in any manner, either directly or indirectly, their skills, training, professional credentials, identity, or services.

Physician assistants shall uphold the doctrine of confidentiality regarding privileged patient information, unless required to release such information by law or such information becomes necessary to protect the welfare of the patient or the community.

Physician assistants shall strive to maintain and increase the quality of individual health care service through individual study and continuing education.

Physician assistants shall have the duty to respect the law, to uphold the dignity of the physician assistant profession and to accept its ethical principles. The physician assistant shall not participate in or conceal any activity that will bring discredit or dishonor to the physician assistant profession and shall expose, without fear or favor, any illegal or unethical conduct in the medical profession.

Physician assistants, ever cognizant of the needs of the community, shall use the knowledge and experience acquired as professionals to contribute to an improved community.

Physician assistants shall place service before material gain and must carefully guard against conflicts of professional interest.

Physician assistants shall strive to maintain a spirit of cooperation with their professional organizations and the general public.

Adopted 1983 House of Delegates; amended 1985 House of Delegates of the American Academy of Physician Assistants.

American Physical Therapy Association Guide for Professional Conduct, Code of Ethics July 1994. Reprinted with permission.

Preamble

This Code of Ethics sets forth ethical principles for the physical therapy profession. Members of this profession are responsible for maintaining and promoting ethical practice. This Code of Ethics, adopted by the American Physical Therapy Association, shall be binding on physical therapists who are members of the Association.

Purpose

This *Guide For Professional Conduc*t (Guide) is intended to serve physical therapists who are members of the American Physical Therapy Association (Association) in interpreting the *Code of Ethics* (Code) and matters of professional conduct. The Guide provides guidelines by which physical therapists may determine the propriety of their conduct. The Code and the Guide apply to all physical therapists who are Association members. These guidelines are subject to changes as the dynamics of the profession change and as new patterns of health care delivery are developed and accepted by the professional community and the public. This Guide is subject to monitoring and timely revision by the Judicial Committee of the Association.

Interpreting Ethical Principles

The interpretations expressed in this Guide are not considered to be all inclusive of situations that could evolve under a specific principle of the Code, but reflect the opinions, decisions, and advice of the Judicial Committee. While the statements of ethical principles apply universally, specific circumstances determine their appropriate application. Input related to current interpretations or situations requiring interpretation is encouraged from Association members.

Principle 1

Physical therapists respect the rights and dignity of all individuals.

1.1 Attitudes of Physical Therapists

A. Physical therapists shall recognize that each individual is different from all other individuals and shall respect and be responsive to those differences.

B. Physical therapists are to be guided at all times by concern for the physical, psychological, and socioeconomic welfare of those individuals entrusted to their care.

C. Physical therapists shall not engage in conduct that constitutes harassment or abuse of colleagues or associates.

1.2 Confidential Information

A. Information relating to the physical therapist-patient relationship is confidential and may not be communicated to a third party not involved in that patient's care without the prior written consent of the patient, subject to applicable law.

B. Information derived from component-sponsored peer review shall be held confidential by the reviewer unless written permission to release the information is obtained from the physical therapist who was reviewed.

C. Information derived from the working relationships of physical therapists shall be held confidential by all parties.

D. Information may be disclosed to appropriate authorities when it is necessary to protect the welfare of an individual or the community. Such disclosure shall be in accordance with applicable law.

Principle 2

Physical therapists comply with the laws and regulations governing the practice of physical therapy.

2.1 Professional Practice

Physical therapists shall provide consultation, evaluation, treatment, and preventive care, in accordance with the laws and regulations of the jurisdiction(s) in which they practice.

Principle 3

Physical therapists accept responsibility for the exercise of sound judgment.

3.1 Acceptance of Responsibility

A. Upon accepting an individual for provision of physical therapy services, physical therapists shall assume the responsibility for evaluating that individual; planning, implementing, and supervising the therapeutic program; reevaluating and changing that program; and maintaining adequate records of the case, including progress reports.

B. When the individual's needs are beyond the scope of the physical therapist's expertise, or when additional services are indicated, the individual shall be so informed and assisted in identifying a qualified provider.

C. Regardless of practice setting, physical therapists shall maintain the ability to make independent judgments.

3.2 Delegation of Responsibility

A. Physical therapists should not delegate to a less qualified person any activity which requires the unique skill, knowledge, and judgment of the physical therapist.

B. The primary responsibility for physical therapy care rendered by supportive personnel rests with the supervising physical therapist. Adequate supervision requires, at a minimum, that a supervising physical therapist perform the following activities:

1. Designate or establish channels of written and oral communication.
2. Interpret available information concerning the individual under care.
3. Provide initial evaluation.
4. Develop plan of care, including short- and long-term goals.
5. Select and delegate appropriate tasks of plan of care.
6. Assess competence of supportive personnel to perform assigned tasks.
7. Direct and supervise supportive personnel in delegated tasks.
8. Identify and document precautions, special problems, contraindications, goals, anticipated progress, and plans for reevaluation.
9. Reevaluate, adjust plan of care when necessary, perform final evaluation, and establish follow-up plan.

3.3 Provision of Services

A. Physical therapists shall recognize the individual's freedom of choice in selection of physical therapy services.

B. Physical therapists' professional practices and their adherence to ethical principles of the Association shall take preference over business practices. Provisions of services for personal financial gain rather than for the need of the individual receiving the services are unethical.

C. When physical therapists judge that an individual will no longer benefit from their services, they shall so inform the individual receiving the services. Physical therapists shall avoid overutilization of their services.

D. In the event of elective termination of physical therapist/patient relationship by the physical therapist, the therapist should take steps to transfer the care of the patient, as appropriate, to another provider.

3.4 Referral Relationships

In a referral situation where the referring practitioner prescribes a treatment program, alteration of that program or extension of physical therapy services beyond that program should be undertaken in consultation with the referring practitioner

3.5 Practice Arrangements

A. Participation in a business, partnership, corporation, or other entity does not exempt the physical therapist, whether employer, partner, or stockholder, either individually or collectively, from the obligation of promoting and maintaining the ethical principles of the Association.

B. Physical therapists shall advise their employer(s) of any employer practice that causes a physical therapist to be in conflict with the ethical principles of the Association. Physical therapist employees shall attempt to rectify aspects of their employment that are in conflict with the ethical principles of the Association.

Principle 4

Physical therapists maintain and promote high standards for physical therapy practice, education, and research.

4.1 Continued Education

A. Physical therapists shall participate in educational activities that enhance their basic knowledge and provide new knowledge.

B. Whenever physical therapists provide continuing education, they shall ensure that course content, objectives, and responsibilities of the instructional faculty are accurately reflected in the promotion of the course.

4.2 Review and Self Assessment

A. Physical therapists shall provide for utilization review of their services.

B. Physical therapists shall demonstrate their commitment to quality assurance by peer review and self assessment.

4.3 Research

A. Physical therapists shall support research activities that contribute knowledge for improved patient care.

B. Physical therapists engaged in research shall ensure:

1. the consent of subjects;
2. confidentiality of the data of individual subjects and the personal identities of the subjects;
3. well-being of all subjects in compliance with facility regulations and laws of the jurisdiction in which the research is conducted;
4. the absence of fraud and plagiarism;
5. full disclosure of support received;
6. appropriate acknowledgement of individuals making a contribution to the research;
7. that animal subjects used in research are treated humanely and in compliance with facility regulations and laws of the jurisdiction in which the research experimentation is conducted.

C. Physical therapists shall report to appropriate authorities any acts in the conduct or presentation of research that appear unethical or illegal.

4.4 Education

A. Physical therapists shall support quality education in academic and clinical settings.

B. Physical therapists functioning in the educational role are responsible to the students, the academic institutions and the clinical settings for promoting ethical conduct in educational activities. Whenever possible, the educator shall ensure:

1. the rights of students in the academic and clinical setting;
2. appropriate confidentiality of personal information;
3. professional conduct toward the student during the academic and clinical processes;
4. assignment to clinical settings prepared to give the student a learning experience.

C. Clinical educators are responsible for reporting to the academic program student conduct which appears to be unethical or illegal.

Principle 5

Physical therapists seek remuneration for their services that is deserved and reasonable.

5.1 Fiscally Sound Remuneration

A. Physical therapists shall never place their own financial interest above the welfare of individuals under their care.

B. Fees for physical therapy services should be reasonable for the service performed, considering the setting in which it is provided, practice costs in the geographic area, judgment of other organizations and other relevant factors.

C. Physical therapists should attempt to ensure that providers, agencies, or other employers adopt physical therapy fee schedules that are reasonable and that encourage access to necessary services.

5.2 Business Practices/Fee Arrangements

A. Physical therapists shall not:

1. directly or indirectly request, receive, or participate in the dividing, transferring, assigning, or rebating of an unearned fee.
2. profit by means of a credit or other valuable consideration, such as an unearned commission, discount, or gratuity in connection with furnishing of physical therapy services.

B. Unless laws impose restrictions to the contrary, physical therapists who provide physical therapy services in a business entity may pool fees and moneys received. Physical therapists may divide or apportion these fees and moneys in accordance with the business agreement.

C. Physical therapists may enter into agreements with organizations to provide physical therapy services if such agreements do not violate the ethical principles of the Association.

5.3 Endorsement of Equipment or Services

A. Physical therapists shall not use influence upon individuals under their care or their families for utilization of equipment or services based upon the direct or indirect financial interest of the physical therapist in such equipment or services. Realizing that these individuals will normally rely on the physical therapists' advice, their best interest must always be maintained as well as their right of free choice relating to the use of any equipment or service. While it cannot be considered unethical for physical therapists to own or have a financial interest in equipment companies, or services, they must act in accordance with law and make full disclosure of their interest whenever such companies or services become the source of equipment or services for individuals under their care.

B. Physical therapists may be remunerated for endorsement or advertisement of equipment or services to the lay public, physical therapists, or other health professionals provided they disclose any financial interest in the production, sale, or distribution of said equipment or services.

C. In endorsing or advertising equipment or services, physical therapists shall use sound professional judgment and shall not give the appearance of Association endorsement.

5.4 Gifts and Other Considerations

A. Physical therapists shall not accept nor offer gifts or other considerations with obligatory conditions attached.

B. Physical therapists shall not accept nor offer gifts or other considerations that affect or give an objective appearance of affecting their professional judgment.

Principle 6

Physical therapists provide accurate information to the consumer about the profession and about those services they provide.

6.1 Information About the Profession

Physical therapists shall endeavor to educate the public to an awareness of the physical therapy profession through such means as publication of articles and participation in seminars, lectures, and civic programs.

6.2 Information About Services

A. Information given to the public shall emphasize that individual problems cannot be treated without individualized evaluations and plans/programs of care.

B. Physical therapists may advertise their services to the public.

C. Physical therapists shall not use, or participate in the use of, any form of communication containing a false, plagiarized, fraudulent, misleading, deceptive, unfair, or sensational statement or claim.

D. A paid advertisement shall be identified as such unless it is apparent from the context that it is a paid advertisement.

Principle 7

Physical therapists accept the responsibility to protect the public and the profession from unethical, incompetent, or illegal acts.

7.1 Consumer Protection

A. Physical therapists shall report any conduct that appears to be unethical, incompetent, or illegal.

B. Physical therapists may not participate in any arrangements in which patients are exploited due to the referring sources enhancing their personal incomes as a result of referring for, prescribing, or recommending physical therapy.

7.2 Disclosure

The physical therapist shall disclose to the patient if the referring practitioner derives compensation from the provision of physical therapy. The physical therapist shall ensure that the individual has freedom of choice in selecting a provider of physical therapy.

Principle 8

Physical therapists participate in efforts to address the health needs of the public.

8.1 Pro Bono Service

Physical therapists should render pro bono publico (reduced or no fee) services to patients lacking the ability to pay for services, as each physical therapist's practice permits.

Issued by Judicial Committee
American Physical Therapy Association
October 1981
Last Amended July 1994

The American Society of Radiologic Technologists Code of Ethics Revised July, 1994. Used with permission.

1. The Radiologic Technologist conducts himself/herself in a professional manner, responds to patient needs and supports colleagues and associates in providing quality patient care.
2. The Radiologic Technologist acts to advance the principle objective of the profession to provide services to humanity with full respect for the dignity of mankind.
3. The Radiologic Technologist delivers patient care and service unrestricted by the concerns of personal attributes or the nature of the disease or illness, and without discrimination, regardless of sex, race, creed, religion, or socioeconomic status.
4. The Radiologic Technologist practices technology founded upon theoretical knowledge and concepts, utilizes equipment and accessories consistent with the purposes for which they have been designed, and employs procedures and techniques appropriately.

5. The Radiologic Technologist assesses situations, exercises care, discretion and judgment, assumes responsibility for professional decisions, and acts in the best interest of the patient.
6. The Radiologic Technologist acts as an agent through observation and communication to obtain pertinent information for the physician to aid in the diagnosis and treatment management of the patient, and recognizes that interpretation and diagnosis are outside the scope of practice for the profession.
7. The Radiologic Technologist utilizes equipment and accessories, employs techniques and procedures, performs services in accordance with an accepted standard of practice, and demonstrates expertise in minimizing the radiation exposure to the patient, self and other members of the health care team.
8. The Radiologic Technologist practices ethical conduct appropriate to the profession, and protects the patient's right to quality radiologic technology care.
9. The Radiologic Technologist respects confidences entrusted in the course of professional practice, respects the patient's right to privacy, and reveals confidential information only as required by law or to protect the welfare of the individual or the community.
10. The Radiologic Technologist continually strives to improve knowledge and skills by participating in educational and professional activities, sharing knowledge with colleagues and investigating new and innovative aspects of professional practice. One means available to improve knowledge and skills is through professional continuing education.

Adopted by: The American Society of Radiologic Technologists
The American Registry of Radiologic Technologists
rev. 7/94

Code of Ethics for Radiation Therapists
August 10, 1994

- The radiation therapist advances the principal objective of the profession to provide services to humanity with full respect for the dignity of mankind.
- The radiation therapist delivers patient care and service unrestricted by concerns of personal attributes or the nature of the disease or illness, and non-discriminatory with respect to race, color, creed, sex, age, disability or national origin.
- The radiation therapist assesses situations; exercises care, discretion and judgment; assumes responsibility for professional decisions; and acts in the best interest of the patient.

- The radiation therapist adheres to the tenets and domains of the *Scope of Practice for Radiation Therapists.*
- The radiation therapist actively engages in lifelong learning to maintain, improve and enhance professional competence and knowledge.

American Association for Respiratory Care Code of Ethics October 22, 1992. Used with permission.

As health care professionals engaged in the performance of respiratory care, respiratory care practitioners must strive, both individually and collectively, to maintain the highest personal and professional standards.

The principles set forth in this document define the basic ethical and moral standards to which each member of the American Association for Respiratory Care should conform.

The respiratory care practitioner shall practice medically acceptable methods of treatment and shall not endeavor to practice beyond his or her competence and the authority given by the physician.

The respiratory care practitioner shall continually strive to increase and improve knowledge and skill and render to each patient the full measure of his or her ability. All services shall be provided with respect for the dignity of the patient, unrestricted by considerations of social or economic status, personal attributes, or the nature of health problems.

The respiratory care practitioner shall be responsible for the competent and efficient performance of the assigned duties and shall expose incompetence and illegal or unethical conduct of members of the profession.

The respiratory care practitioner shall hold in strict confidence all privileged information concerning the patient and refer all inquiries to the physician in charge of the patient's medical care.

The respiratory care practitioner shall not accept gratuities for preferential consideration of the patient and shall guard against conflicts of interest.

The respiratory care practitioner shall uphold the dignity and honor of the profession and abide by its ethical principles. The practitioner should be familiar with existing state and federal laws governing the practice of respiratory care and comply with those laws.

The respiratory care practitioner shall cooperate with other health care professionals and participate in activities to promote community and national efforts to meet the health needs of the public.

The American Speech-Language-Hearing Association Code of Ethics 1994 version. Reprinted by permission.

Preamble

The preservation of the highest standards of integrity and ethical principles is vital to the responsible discharge of obligations in the professions of speech-language pathology and audiology. This Code of Ethics sets forth the fundamental principles and rules considered essential to this purpose.

Every individual who is (a) a member of the American Speech-Language-Hearing Association, whether certified or not, (b) a nonmember holding the Certificate of Clinical Competence from the Association, (c) an applicant for membership or certification, or (d) a Clinical Fellow seeking to fulfill standards for certification shall abide by this Code of Ethics.

Any action that violates the spirit and purpose of this Code shall be considered unethical. Failure to specify any particular responsibility or practice in this Code of Ethics shall not be construed as denial of the existence of such responsibilities or practices.

The fundamentals of ethical conduct are described by Principles of Ethics and by Rules of Ethics as they relate to responsibility to persons served, to the public, and to the professions of speech-language pathology and audiology.

Principles of Ethics, aspirational and inspirational in nature, form the underlying moral basis for the Code of Ethics. Individuals shall observe these principles as affirmative obligations under all conditions of professional activity.

Rules of Ethics are specific statements of minimally acceptable professional conduct or of prohibitions and are applicable to all individuals.

Principle of Ethics I

Individuals shall honor their responsibility to hold paramount the welfare of persons they serve professionally.

Rules of Ethics

A. Individuals shall provide all services competently.
B. Individuals shall use every resource, including referral when appropriate, to ensure that high-quality service is provided.
C. Individuals shall not discriminate in the delivery of professional services on the basis of race, sex, age, religion, national origin, sexual orientation, or handicapping condition.

D. Individuals shall fully inform the persons they serve of the nature and possible effects of services rendered and products dispensed.
E. Individuals shall evaluate the effectiveness of services rendered and of products dispensed and shall provide services or dispense products only when benefit can reasonably be expected.
F. Individuals shall not guarantee the results of any treatment or procedure, directly or by implications; however, they may make a reasonable statement of prognosis.
G. Individuals shall not evaluate or treat speech, language, or hearing disorders solely by correspondence.
H. Individuals shall maintain adequate records of professional services rendered and products dispensed and shall allow access to these records when appropriately authorized.
I. Individuals shall not reveal, without authorization, any professional or personal information about the person served professionally, unless required by law to do so, or unless doing so is necessary to protect the welfare of the person or of the community.
J. Individuals shall not charge for services not rendered, nor shall they misrepresent[1], in any fashion, services rendered or products dispensed.
K. Individuals shall use persons in research or as subjects of teaching demonstrations only with their informed consent.
L. Individuals shall withdraw from professional practice when substance abuse or an emotional or mental disability may adversely affect the quality of services they render.

Principle of Ethics II

Individuals shall honor their responsibility to achieve and maintain the highest level of professional competence.

Rules of Ethics

A. Individuals shall engage in the provision of clinical services only when they hold the appropriate Certificate of Clinical Competence or when they are in the certification process and are supervised by an individual who holds the appropriate Certificate of Clinical Competence.
B. Individuals shall engage in only those aspects of the professions that are within the scope of their competence, considering their level of education, training, and experience.
C. Individuals shall continue their professional development throughout their careers.

[1]For purposes of this Code of Ethics, misrepresentation includes any untrue statements or statements that are likely to mislead. Misrepresentation also includes the failure to state any information that is material and that ought, in fairness, to be considered.

D. Individuals shall delegate the provision of clinical services only to persons who are certified or to persons in the education or certification process who are appropriately supervised. The provision of support services may be delegated to persons who are neither certified nor in the certification process only when a certificate holder provides appropriate supervision.
E. Individuals shall prohibit any of their professional staff from providing services that exceed the staff member's competence, considering the staff member's level of education, training, and experience.
F. Individuals shall ensure that all equipment used in the provision of services is in proper working order and is properly calibrated.

Principle of Ethics III

Individuals shall honor their responsibility to the public by promoting public understanding of the professions, by supporting the development of services designed to fulfill the unmet needs of the public, and by providing accurate information in all communications involving any aspect of the professions.

Rules of Ethics

A. Individuals shall not misrepresent their credentials, competence, education, training, or experience.
B. Individuals shall not participate in professional activities that constitute a conflict of interest.
C. Individuals shall not misrepresent diagnostic information, services rendered, or products dispensed or engage in any scheme or artifice to defraud in connection with obtaining payment or reimbursement for such services or products.
D. Individuals' statements to the public shall provide accurate information about the nature and management of communication disorders, about the professions, and about professional services.
E. Individuals' statements to the public—advertising, announcing, and marketing their professional services, reporting research results, and promoting products—shall adhere to prevailing professional standards and shall not contain misrepresentations.

Principle of Ethics IV

Individuals shall honor their responsibilities to the professions and their relationships with colleagues, students, and members of allied professions. Individuals shall uphold the dignity and autonomy of the professions, maintain harmonious interprofessional and intraprofessional relationships, and accept the professions' self-imposed standards.

Rules of Ethics

A. Individuals shall prohibit anyone under their supervision from engaging in any practice that violates the Code of Ethics.

B. Individuals shall not engage in dishonesty, fraud, deceit, misrepresentation, or any form of conduct that adversely reflects on the professions or on the individual's fitness to serve persons professionally.
C. Individuals shall assign credit only to those who have contributed to a publication, presentation, or product. Credit shall be assigned in proportion to the contribution and only with the contributor's consent.
D. Individuals' statements to colleagues about professional services, research results, and products shall adhere to prevailing professional standards and shall contain no misrepresentations.
E. Individuals shall not provide professional services without exercising independent professional judgment, regardless of referral source or prescription.
F. Individuals who have reason to believe that the Code of Ethics has been violated shall inform the Ethical Practice Board.
G. Individuals shall cooperate fully with the Ethical Practice Board in its investigation and adjudication of matters related to this Code of Ethics.

GLOSSARY OF TERMS

A priori: derived from self-evident proposition

Absolutism: the view that there is a single, universal standard of reference for deciding morality

Act-based theory: a kind of action theory in which principles are applied directly to individual actions

Action theory: a theory of right action in which general principles are articulated, sometimes through the use of rules, in order to make moral evaluations of actions (rather than the character of the actors); cf. virtue theory

Antinomianism: the position that ethical actions must be evaluated in each situation without the use of any rules or guidelines; cf. legalism, rules of practice, situationalism

Autonomy: the governing of one's self according to one's own system of morals and beliefs or lifeplan

Avoidance of killing: the principle that actions (or rules) are morally right insofar as they do not involve killing or wrong insofar as they do involve killing

Beneficence: the state of doing or producing good; cf. nonmaleficence. Also the moral principle that actions are right insofar as they produce good

Best interest standard: judgment based on an idea of what would be most beneficial to a patient; cf. substituted judgment

Consequentialism: the normative theory that the rightness or wrongness of actions is determined by anticipated or known consequences, cf. deontologism

Contract: a term sometimes used to describe the fiduciary relationship in professional ethics grounded in promises or pledges

Covenant: a solemn agreement between two or more parties that, as related to health care, emphasizes the moral and social character of the bond between professional and patient

Cultural relativism: the view that moral judgments are grounded only in each culture's collective opinion

De facto: in reality, actual; cf. de jure

De jure: by right, by law; cf. de facto

Deontologism: a theory according to which actions are judged right or wrong based upon inherent right-making characteristics or principles rather than on their consequences

Descriptive relativism: the claim that different cultures have differing views as to which matters are believed to be moral

Distributive justice: the just allocation of society's benefits and burdens

Double effect: the doctrine that an evil effect is morally acceptable provided a proportional good effect will accrue, evil is not intended, the evil effect is not the means to the good, and the action is not intrinsically evil

Due process criterion: a criterion sometimes used to justify paternalism by which the individual who coerces paternalistically must have observed proper procedure and have proper authorization

Duty proper: a duty decided after taking into account all relevant principles and applying some theory of how to reconcile conflict among principles

Egalitarianism: a social philosophy or principle that advocates human equality

Elements of consent: the categories of information that may be included in an informed consent (such as the benefits, the harms, the alternative treatments, the costs, etc.)

Emotivism: the view that ethical utterances evince emotions rather than make cognitive claims

Empirical absolutism: a type of absolutism that has some empirical foundation; the view that there is a single, universal standard of reference that is an empirical phenomenon such as the law of nature

Ethical: an evaluation of actions, rules, or the character of persons, especially as it refers to the examination of a systematic theory of rightness or wrongness at the ultimate level

Fidelity: the state of being faithful, which includes obligations of loyalty and the keeping of promises and commitments. Also the principle that actions are right insofar as they demonstrate such loyalty

Fiduciary relation: a relationship based on trust and confidence that commitments made between parties will be honored

Formalism: the view that actions are right or wrong based on their formal characteristics rather than their consequences (often a synonym for deontologism)

Guiding rules: (guidelines) *See* rules of thumb

Human immunodeficiency virus (HIV): a retrovirus responsible for acquired immune deficiency syndrome (AIDS)

Intuitionism: the view that moral knowledge is known intuitively rather than by revelation, empirical knowledge, reason, or some other way

Justice: (1) a moral principle that holds that actions (or rules) are morally right insofar as they reflect a specified pattern of distribution of benefits and harms; (2) a synonym for moral rightness; right taking into account all moral principles

Legalism: the position that ethical action consists in strict conformity to law or rules; cf. antinomianism, rules of practice, situationalism

Limits of reasonableness: the limits to which a surrogate decision may go and still be tolerable to one who insists that such decisions be reasonable

Mature minor: someone who is legally a minor, but who possesses sufficient capacity for autonomy to be treated as a substantially autonomous decision maker

Metaethics: the branch of ethics having to do with the meaning, justification, or grounding of ethical claims; cf. normative

Metaphysical: the principles underlying a particular subject or system of beliefs about the nature of reality

Microallocation: distribution of resources on a small scale

Moral: an evaluation of actions or the character of persons, especially as it refers to ad hoc judgments by individuals or society

Neutralism: a characteristic of moral or ethical evaluations in which there is general application not favoring one party

Noncognitivism: the view that ethical propositions are not cognitive propositions (cf. emotivism; prescriptivism)

Nonnaturalism: the view that ethical phenomena are not natural properties

Nontherapeutic: something that does not serve the purposes of benefiting an individual patient

Nonmaleficence: the state of not doing harm or evil; cf. beneficence. Also the moral principle that actions are right insofar as they avoid producing harm or evil

Normative: the branch of ethics having to do with which actions are right or wrong, which states are valuable, or which character traits of persons are praiseworthy; cf. metaethics

Normative relativism: the claim that there is no single universal foundation of moral judgments

Ordering: a characteristic of moral or ethical evaluations on which a set of principles, rules, or character assessments provides a basis for ranking conflicting claims

Paternalism: the system of action in which one person treats another the way a father treats a child striving to promote the other's good even against the other's wishes

Personal relativism: the claim that a behavior or character is good or right that conforms to one's personal standard of goodness or rightness

Prescriptivism: the view that ethical utterances function to prescribe conduct rather than make cognitive claims

***Prima facie* duty:** a duty based on consideration of a single moral dimension of an action represented by one moral principle; cf. duty proper

Professional standard for consent: the standard that health professionals must disclose all information that their professional colleagues similarly situated would disclose about a proposed procedure; cf. reasonable person standard, subjective standard

Publicity: a characteristic of moral or ethical evaluations in which one must be willing to state the evaluation and the basis on which it is made publicly

Reasonable person standard of consent: the duty of health professionals to disclose all information that a reasonable person would find meaningful in making a decision whether to consent to a proposed procedure; cf. professional standard, subjective standard

Rigorism: the view that moral rules should be applied relatively rigidly (see also legalism; cf. antinomianism)

Rule-based theory: a kind of action theory in which rules, rather than acts, are used to apply principles to individual actions

Rule-utilitarianism: a version of utilitarianism that assesses actions according to the benefits and harms of alternative rules or systems of rules; see also situational utilitarianism

Rules of practice: rules that define general practices in a society; the position that ethical action must be judged by such rules rather than by direct assessment of individual cases; cf. antinomianism, legalism, situationalism

Rules of thumb: the view that rules merely summarize past moral judgments (see also summary rules, guiding rules, rules of practice, antinomianism, legalism)

Secular ethics: theories of what is good and bad, or right or wrong, based on criteria other than religious doctrine

Situationalism: **a.** a version of utilitarianism that assesses actions according to the benefits and harms of the individual action, that is situationally; see also act-based theory
b. the position that ethical action must be judged in each situation guided by, but not directly determined by, rules; cf. antinomianism, rules of practice

Social relativism: the view that moral judgments are grounded only in each society's collective opinion (cf. cultural relativism)

Strong paternalism: the provision of treatment for the good of an individual against the wishes of the individual who is known to be substantially autonomous

Subjective standard of consent: the standard that health professionals must disclose the information that the individual patient needs in making a decision whether to consent to a proposed procedure; cf. professional standard, reasonable person standard

Substituted judgment standard: judgment based on an idea of what the patient would have wanted considering his or her beliefs and values; cf. best interest standard

Summary rules: the view that rules merely summarize past moral judgments (see also rules of thumb; cf. rules of practice, antinomianism, legalism)

Standards of consent: the frame of reference upon which a consent may be evaluated (see reasonable person standard, professional standard, subjective standard)

Theological absolutism: a type of absolutism in which the absolute or universal standard of reference in ethics is a deity

Theological universalism: a type of universalism in which the absolute or universal standard of reference in ethics is a deity

Ultimacy: a characteristic of moral or ethical evaluations that they are grounded in the highest standard by which one might judge

Universality: a characteristic of moral or ethical evaluations in which an action or character trait should be evaluated the same by all people

Utilitarianism: the view that an action is deemed morally acceptable because it produces the greatest balance of good over evil taking into account all individuals affected

Utility: the state of being useful or producing good

Value theory: a theory of which objects or states are rationally desirable; what counts as a good or a harm

Veracity: the principle that actions (or rules) are morally right insofar as they involve telling the truth and wrong insofar as they involve lying

Virtue theory: a theory that focuses on the character traits of the actor rather than the ethics of the behavior itself; cf. action theory

Weak paternalism: the provision of treatment against the wishes of individuals whose autonomy is compromised

INDEX

B

C

D

E

X